"No child should ever have [...] ice, whatever its source. Debra A [...] ope. I urge anyone who has a chi [...] ma to read this book immediately."

—Clau [...] ., author of It Will
Never Happen to Me

"*Children Changed by Trauma* is a wonderful book that blends what we know about the effects of trauma with first hand accounts. I believe the book will help parents and teachers better understand children's traumatic experiences. There is also much here that will assist adults in learning about their own early experiences with trauma. This is an important and relevant book as we begin to acknowledge how trauma can shape our past and our future."

—Marleen Wong, Director of Mental Health
Services District Crisis Teams, Los Angeles
Unified School District

"*Children Changed by Trauma* offers good, sound advice to child-care practitioners. The book is easy to follow and comprehensive and provides a personal touch with the incorporation of real-life experiences. This is a must read for anyone who works with children in trauma."

—Krista R. Flannigan, J.D, and Robin F.
Finegan, M.A., Victim Services Consultants,
Idaho Springs and Denver Colorado

"Unfortunately children's lives today often include exposure to, or involvement in traumatic events. In this practical and user-friendly book, Dr. Alexander offers the parents of these children workable strategies to help their children recover from these traumas. Using the framework of trauma theory as a template, Dr. Alexander gives concrete case examples and interventions that can be explored both immediately or long after an event. Also a valuable resource for therapists, teachers, pastors and others, this book is designed to be used, and use it I will! I urge potential readers to do the same."

—Mary Beth Williams, Ph.D., CTS, LCSW,
President, Association of Traumatic Stress
Specialists

"This book will soothe and inspire the parents of traumatized children. It is full of the kind of intelligent, compassionate, and clearly written advice that truly fosters healing. Dr. Alexander draws on both her professional and personal experiences to illuminate the issues, and the accounts of real-life trauma that she documents make the book particularly valuable. Her practical suggestions are a gold mine and will help children and adults grow strong again and regain humor, peace, and joy."

> —Jennifer J. Freyd, Ph.D., Professor of Psychology, University of Oregon, and author of *Betrayal Trauma: The Logic of Forgetting Abuse*

"This powerful and useful book comes from an author with years of experience in the field. She boils down complex concepts and jargon-heavy theory into clear and concise methods of working with children who have survived a trauma. *Children Changed by Trauma* helps us all become more sensitive to traumatized children. Parents, friends, teachers and counselors stand to benefit from its lucidity."

> —Charles R. Figley, Ph.D., Professor and Director, Florida State University Traumatology Institute

Children
CHANGED
by
TRAUMA

a healing guide

Debra Whiting Alexander, Ph.D.

New Harbinger Publications, Inc.

Publisher's Note

This publication is designed to provide accurate and authoritative information in regard to the subject matter covered. It is sold with the understanding that the publisher is not engaged in rendering psychological, financial, legal, or other professional services. If expert assistance or counseling is needed, the services of a competent professional should be sought.

Distributed in the U.S.A. by Publishers Group West; in Canada by Raincoast Books; in Great Britain by Airlift Book Company, Ltd.; in South Africa by Real Books, Ltd.; in Australia by Boobook; and in New Zealand by Tandem Press.

Copyright © 1999 by Debra Whiting Alexander, Ph.D.
New Harbinger Publications, Inc.
5674 Shattuck Avenue
Oakland, CA 94609

Cover design © 1999 by Lightbourne Images
Edited by Angela Watrous
Text design by Tracy Marie Powell

Library of Congress Catalog Card Number: 99-74369
ISBN 1-57224-166-7 Paperback

New Harbinger Publications' Website address: www.newharbinger.com

01   00   99
10   9   8   7   6   5   4   3   2   1

First printing

Contents

Dedication

To all the children on these pages whom I have had the honor to know and love. It is through their eyes that this book began and from their hearts that the stories are told.

To Debora Jean Martin, for surviving and taking the path to healing with me.

To parents and adults everywhere for taking the path to healing with their children.

Preface

When I was seven, I went to an air show with my family. Thousands of people had gathered and crowds of us were walking over a wide-open rocky dirt terrain. Ahead were old railroad tracks to cross before we reached the observation field where the show was to take place.

It was a hot, Sunday afternoon, like most I grew up with in San Diego. I remember seeing adults around me wearing fancy church clothes, but most of my steps were focused on the new pair of white buckled sandals I was so pleased to be wearing. I carefully navigated them over the unavoidable stones and around dry crusty ditches, trying to keep the dust off of them.

I almost lost my balance every time I looked up at the city of grown-ups around me. They hovered like giant skyscrapers, swaying against the sky. It was much easier to focus on the twelve inches directly in front of my feet. One time when I looked ahead to see how much closer we were to the railroad tracks, an ancient-looking woman off to my right caught my attention.

She was wearing a dark purple-and-lavender flowered chiffon dress. I noticed her because she reminded me of a bedspread we had at home. She wore a hat that had fake flowers on the side of it. A small purse hung on her wrist, which was covered by a white glove. Everything matched. I had never seen anything like it. More importantly, I had never seen anyone who looked like our bedspread before.

And then she lost her balance and fell. I had been looking at her shoes when it happened. I watched her step gingerly over the same ditches I was having trouble with when she suddenly became stiff and awkward. No one was able to catch her in time. I saw her head hit the metal track we were quickly approaching. The sound startled me. Something about it was very wrong.

Once she landed, she didn't move. The grown-ups around her let out a horrified gasp and rushed to her side. One lady screamed so loud I thought she was falling, too. They sounded so scared and worried that I became frightened. I felt my heart beat faster than I could count.

Two men dressed in white pants and shirts carried the woman in the purple dress away. They put her on a shiny silver stretcher with a white sheet across it, and then they disappeared. I was perplexed. This frail old woman, who just moments earlier had been sharing the same kind of day I was having, was gone. We were going to watch the same show and stand on the same field to do the same thing. I couldn't understand how she could be there one minute and gone the next. Hurt and dying, just that quick. No one was able to tell me if she would be okay or why it happened. Everyone kept walking forward. I tried to turn around to see where she went, twisting my neck until it hurt. But it was no use. I only saw swarms of legs marching forward, certain to trample me if I didn't keep up.

After that, I didn't feel happy anymore. Not even at the sight of my sandals. I only remember hanging on tighter to the hand holding mine, so it wouldn't happen to me.

I'm told I watched the air show and saw famous planes performing spectacular maneuvers over a cheering crowd. I remember nothing more of that day than the old woman in the purple-flowered dress, who in an instant was hurled over a track and lay lifeless on the ground.

I worried about her for a long time, and on some level I suppose I have continued my concern for her over the course of my life. I never cross a set of railroad tracks without remembering her.

I often give the woman in the purple-flowered dress some of the credit for my training as a writer. Trauma does in a moment what writers spend a lifetime trying to do. It causes you to pay attention. The senses are heightened. Images, thoughts, feelings, smells, and a myriad of memories are recorded somewhere deep inside. Vivid details are preserved for safekeeping until they can be digested.

These moments are sacred, because in their own way they touch the soul.

For the writer, the experience must be properly placed on paper. For the trauma survivor, it's an experience that must be integrated into life. Having done both, I know it is the trauma survivor who carries the enormous burden of bringing the experience back to life—so it can be put to rest. Children and adults who have experienced trauma can be tormented by what they went through or find meaning through their suffering and be strengthened. With some thanks due to the woman in the purple-flowered dress, this book is about helping children find meaning and strength.

—*Debra Whiting Alexander, Ph.D., LMFT, CTS*

Acknowledgments

Writing this book was a labor of love. Several "midwives" assisted me along the way. Thank you to Janice Carr, Susan Jorgensen, Corinne Marie, and Donna Yates for encouragement and refreshing insight.

I thank the staff of the Center for Community Counseling in Eugene, Oregon, for their generous enthusiasm and support for my work, especially Nowell King, Victoria Scott, and Nancy Weisel.

I gratefully acknowledge the work of Alice Miller, M.D., whose contributions have influenced my life both personally and professionally.

I am indebted to all the children, families, and adults I have had the honor of working with over the years. I have been enriched by being a witness to their growth and healing.

I thank my parents for sharing a spiritual foundation with me that I will carry always. And to my sister, Sherie Whiting, who shares my childhood experiences as no one else can.

To New Harbinger Publications, and especially to my editor Angela Watrous, heartfelt appreciation for your clarity and vision in bringing this book to life. It has been a privilege to work with all of you.

I am especially grateful for my friend, Kathryn Wilson, who encouraged and strengthened this book from its beginnings with her valuable input, steady wisdom, and unwavering support. Thank you for being the friend I always need.

Thank you to RCA (Bob) for the gift of your love.

And finally, my deepest thanks go to my daughter, Katelyn Jenne, who inspires me.

Introduction

My family is not unusual. We live in a relatively safe neighborhood, share the friendship of good neighbors, and live an average middle-class life. However, by the age of seven my daughter was aware of murder, shootings, and child abuse. Our family had been victimized by a destructive burglary in our home, and my daughter had seen prostitution on our streets and witnessed a physical assault in the parking lot of our local grocery store. Despite my best efforts to protect and minimize my daughter's exposure to trauma, the world continued to roll a parade of tragedies before her eyes.

Today, all children are at risk. They are bombarded regularly by news of senseless tragedies. The media as well as real-life scenarios on the streets are packed with images that have the power to evoke anxiety beyond what most children are able to handle on their own. Children have a limited capacity to absorb this toxic part of life.

An increasing number of children are being more directly impacted by crime and trauma. They are the targeted victims, the loved ones of victims, and the innocent bystanders of random acts of crime and violence. They are also the survivors of community-wide disasters and traumatic events. Some children have witnessed unspeakable acts of violence in their own schools. Others witness it regularly in their homes. These children are forever changed. What they have learned is that life is not safe.

When trauma hits, it is usually sudden. It may be an act of human cruelty, such as a crime spree, or it may be a car or plane crash, a sudden or untimely death, or a natural disaster like a tornado, earthquake, or hurricane. It can happen in seconds. Trauma abruptly rips you out of the comfort and safety of your life and thrusts you into the depths of loss and despair. Children are totally unprepared for these experiences in life. Most parents are unsure of how to help their children through such intense psychological, emotional, and spiritual injuries.

How do you respond to your children's questions when they ask why something happened or if it will happen again? When children look to you for answers and seek your reassurance, what can you say? They want to understand and know they're safe, and they want answers. Most of all, your children look to you to regain a sense of hope when the world has turned crazy and hopeless.

This book cannot offer you a detour around suffering, but it can offer you a path and direction through it. It also cannot take the place of therapy. Professional help is needed for most, if not all, children and their families following a traumatic event. Still, much successful healing work can and does happen through parents and other adults children love and trust. The relationship you share can be the strongest link in the chain of their healing.

Witnessing violence and trauma affects a child's whole being: the heart, mind, body, and soul. Each of these parts demands healing. If wounds are not tended, the effects may last a lifetime. Untreated, trauma can even lead some children on the path to personal violence in the future.

Throughout each chapter of this book I have described case examples of children exposed to trauma. By illustrating their experiences, I will help you understand the impact of trauma, become familiar with the normal responses children are likely to experience, and give you specific ways to help your child feel whole again. Step by step, you will journey through the heart, mind, body, and soul of children who have healed—and see how they did it. For recovery to be complete, I believe it is the soul that lies at the root of trauma resolution. You will also read about the important role humor can play in your child's healing process.

What I have written is a blend of my clinical experience as a child therapist and my personal experience as a mother. The majority of the case descriptions are from my work, but the personal insights also come from resolving the impact of crime in my own family. Names and identifying details have been changed to protect confidentiality of clients involved.

Trauma does change all who encounter it. For the survivors, life will never be the same. This does not mean life is over or that life will be worse—it simply means it will be different. The joy and innocence your child once enjoyed will return, but healing is a process that happens in unique ways to each person. You can use this book to help expand the love, wisdom, and knowledge you already possess, enhancing your ability to help your child through this process.

While trauma has the potential to tear families apart, the recovery process can also bond families together. By helping your children find meaning and strength in times of tragedy, they can gain a new appreciation for life and for those who love them. It is my hope that the information you find in this book will support the individual recovery and healing of your child, as well as strengthen your family relationship in new and meaningful ways.

Finally, it is important to note that healing cannot begin until you and your children are physically safe and protected. If you are experiencing violence in your home or feel threatened in any way, seek help and support immediately. Call the police, a local shelter, or a counseling center for assistance. *No one* deserves to be abused, threatened, or treated unkindly. You and your family have the right to live in a safe home. Your lives may depend on it. Domestic violence is a crime. Confidential information and help is available (see Resources at the end of this book).

If you are concerned that you may be mistreating or abusing a child or that you may be at risk for hurting a child, confidential information and help is available (see Resources at the end of this book).

Part I

Facilitating Your Child's Healing

1

Healing the Heart

"It hurts inside and out."

It was the middle of the day, a hot and humid afternoon, when Maria witnessed the brutal murder of her baby-sitter, a woman whom Maria loved deeply. They had just sat down together on the front porch steps with root-beer floats when an angry man approached them with a knife.

Moments later, at the tender age of eight, Maria watched the man—in uncontrollable fury—stab her baby-sitter over thirty times. Maria stood in shock as her baby-sitter lay dying before her eyes. Maria saw her baby-sitter's body twitch as blood poured from her chest. She watched tears streaming down her baby-sitter's cheeks as she lay gasping for air in pools of blood. Overcome by terror, Maria managed to run from the scene, fearing she would be his next victim. Maria ran, but later struggled with a sense of profound shame for having "left" her baby-sitter behind. Maria was haunted by the memory of her baby-sitter's face when their eyes met for the last time.

In the weeks following the murder, Maria became mute. She was the only witness to the crime and detectives on the case were anxious to hear her story. She refused to talk to anyone. Maria and her mother were referred to my office for help.

This young girl taught me many things. The first thing I learned from Maria was that I needed to be able to be mute, too.

We spent many sessions sitting in a rocking chair together,
saying nothing. Sometimes we rocked and sometimes we sat still.
I remember Maria's hands, because we spent hours examining them
together. Sometimes she would twist a small piece of her clothing,
wringing it tightly. Most of the time, however, her hands did not
move. Her body sank limply into the chair and I could see the effort
it took her to lift even one finger.

I told Maria that I didn't blame her for being quiet. I told her
I believed she would talk again when she was ready. I let her know
I felt confident that she would eventually talk like she used to and
that she would know when it was the right time to do so. I said
I understood why it would be hard to talk about what she saw.
I let her know that I would listen to whatever she wanted to say.
I explained that when she was ready, telling me about what
happened would help her feel better again.

The detective made daily visits to my office, hoping for a
"breakthrough." Every day he asked when I thought she'd be ready
to talk. I continued to disappoint him; my response was always the
same: "She'll tell me what she wants to when she's ready, and I don't
have a clue when that will be." Given enough time, I hoped Maria
would come to trust me, but the only thing I was certain of was
that Maria was the only one who could decide when she would tell
her story.

One day in a session with Maria, I wondered aloud what the
detective would do if both of us refused to answer his questions.
I suggested to Maria that we invite the "pesky" detective in and say
nothing together. She spoke her first word to me at last: "Okay."

The detective eagerly entered my office, hope written all over
his face. He gently explained what he needed to know. He said he
needed Maria to tell the story of what happened so he could "put
this bad man away where he could never hurt anyone again."
I sensed his urgency and impatience, and I knew he was right to
be asking. He wanted a conviction. For a moment, I imagined joining
his efforts to coach the information out of her, a fleeting thought
sparked by my own contempt for the killer.

The detective grew increasingly uncomfortable with our lack of
response to his questions and comments. I finally told him, "We're
not talking." Maria and I exchanged a knowing look. We shared a
secret now. After he left Maria let out a short giggle. No words or
sentences, but it was a sound full of meaning just the same. Trust
could start to build now.

Maria and I continued to see each other almost every day.

I was grateful every time she stepped through my door, fearing she would grow tired of our appointments before I could help. I told her I liked talking to her even though she still said nothing. One day I asked if she'd be willing to pretend to be my counselor and listen to me talk. I invited her to help me out if I was stuck for words or if I said something she thought wasn't quite right. I told her she could tell me in any way she wanted—by nodding, writing, or using gestures. I began to describe my feelings about what happened to her. I told Maria how sorry I was. I explained the sadness I felt for what she saw and remembered. Thirty seconds later Maria began talking. With hands pushed against her chest, she said, "It hurts inside and out. It hurts in my heart."

Her pain, at last, had a voice. We had connected.

I wanted to embrace her, this delicate yet resilient being. She was so fragile that I was afraid she would shatter if I did. She wrapped her arms around my waist and began to cry. Her feelings finally could be shared. I was able to comfort her.

Maria had a wound so deep it penetrated her heart. In the weeks ahead I learned just how powerful a medicine love would be for her traumatic pain. The healing process could not begin without it.

Trauma Hurts the Heart

Bearing witness to a tragic event is painful. Like Maria, children often hold their hands over their hearts when they show "where it hurts most." It is normal to attach feelings and emotions to the heart. When asked to draw what they feel, many traumatized children draw pictures of broken or blackened hearts.

The pain and heartbreak children feel is complicated by troubling symptoms of stress and fear. In this state of emotional turmoil, children who have been profoundly impacted by trauma often say they feel like they're "going crazy."

The Emotional Balancing Act

Parents and children cope with stress on a daily basis. Lost car keys, a teacher conference, waking up late for work or school, or even something as simple as breaking a glass disrupts a normal routine. Stressful experiences throw you off balance, if even for a few moments.

The majority of people handle the day-to-day stresses that interrupt their lives relatively easily. They regain their balance or sense of emotional equilibrium and usually the rest of the day continues unaffected. But when something traumatic happens, it throws you so far out of balance and out of the normal range of your equilibrium that it is impossible to regain it (Young 1998). I've heard children describe the experience by saying, "I feel like I'm in a nightmare, but I'm not waking up."

The effects of trauma can put children on an emotional roller coaster. One day they're sad, the next day nervous, another day it's forgotten, the next day it's all they think about. Some children say they feel as if they're walking on a tight rope and can't catch their balance. They fear life will fall apart again at any given moment. The ups and downs and anxiety of living on the edge take an emotional toll. Given enough stress, no one is immune to these effects.

When emotional balance is lost, children do not behave, think, act, or feel the same. And how could they? Their lives have shifted out of kilter. You can help them learn ways to find their balance again and hold it. This is how to start:

- Assure children that having frightening or confusing feelings does not mean they are "going crazy." What happened was crazy, but they are not.

- Explain to children that as strange as it may sound, part of what will help them feel better is to let themselves feel out of balance for a while.

- Tell them it's not wrong, bad, or weak to feel the way they do.

- Explain that the way they feel is the same for most kids and adults after an experience like theirs.

- Let them know it is important for them to accept help and support for a while until they feel more like themselves.

- Reassure them that while right now it might take effort and concentration to get normal things done, getting their balance will become easier the more they do it (just like learning to ride a bike).

Like adults, with adequate support and care children will regain their sense of emotional equilibrium. However, when it comes back, it will be in a different place. Children will never be the same. This does not mean life will be worse, it means it will be *different*. Some children even grow stronger with the new balance they acquire.

Trauma changes you. As one child said, "This changed me forever. It's changed everyone who saw it. I don't know how I'll feel ten years from now, but I know I'll be different than I would've been—all because of this."

Depression

When the world falls apart, the shock immediately following the experience can soon give way to depression. Children experience depression in different ways. They can be subdued and withdrawn, becoming mute like Maria, or they can be irritable and explosive, seeming angry rather than sad. The despair children sometimes feel over what they've witnessed or experienced can be so overwhelming that they may need to find ways to forget what they saw. Children may do this by telling you they don't remember or don't want to talk about it. They may also:

- change the subject when it's discussed
- practice behaviors that distract themselves or you from their feelings
- express anger and irritability with you or others
- say it was "no big deal"
- refuse to say anything at all

What You Can Say to Help

Sometimes it's hard to know what to say, but the way you respond to your child's feelings of despair is important. You can offer comfort and support by saying what you feel. Here are some ideas to help you get started:

- I'm sorry it happened.
- I'm glad you're safe.
- Hearts can hurt the same way a broken bone does. Hurting is part of the cure.
- Broken hearts do heal.
- You can't forget or stop the pain because this is something too painful to forget.
- It's normal to feel sad at a time like this.
- Crying over something sad is not the same as acting like a baby.

- People do not die from crying.

- Feelings may change from day to day. You may also feel a lot of different ways at once.

- Feelings can be confusing to people who have been through what you have.

- You can trust your feelings.

- No one can make the pain disappear.

- You can never completely forget what happened, but with time it will feel less frightening to remember.

- You may allow yourself to forget for a while, but you shouldn't be surprised if you get upset when something reminds you.

- It's okay to remember.

- Remembering won't always feel this hard.

- I can see you feel very angry/sad/scared right now. How can I help?

- Let's think of ways you can help yourself feel better (or safer).

- Draw a picture of what you can do to help yourself feel better (or safer).

- Friends, family, counselors, and others can help you learn ways to live with what happened.

- I can listen, even when what you say is sad or hard to share. No matter what you say, I'll always love you.

Your child's sadness may look different from day to day. It may remain constant or not seem obvious at all. Children may be tearful, withdrawn, angry, or depressed. They may appear emotionally "numb." They may exhibit increased energy or decreased energy. Some people notice that their children move in and out of all these symptoms very quickly. Others notice an ongoing pattern of the same predictable behaviors.

Trauma Affects Self-Esteem

Children who carry strong feelings of self-worth and feel good about themselves are generally more hopeful about life. However, self-esteem can take a beating when tragedy strikes. The self-confidence your child once enjoyed may be temporarily buried beneath the emotional rubble that trauma often leaves behind.

The mixed emotions that children are sorting through often interfere with the view they once had of themselves. They may question their strengths and abilities, the same way they now question their sense of security and safety in the world. Self-esteem can be impacted by feelings of guilt or self-blame for what happened. It may cause children to struggle with feelings of self-doubt if they were unable to do the "right" thing under pressure or duress at the time of the incident.

Children may be too fearful, anxious, or sad to approach life with their usual level of energy and enthusiasm. They may stop taking the healthy risks they need in order to feel good about themselves (Krupnick and Horowitz 1980). When children stop trying new skills, expanding their interests, or joining new groups, they lose two important self-esteem builders: the experience of success and accomplishment. Consequently, feelings of self-worth diminish and self-esteem suffers.

Rebuilding Confidence and Self-Worth

You can help change your child's outlook and emotional state by nurturing his or her feelings of confidence and self-worth. Self-esteem nurtures feelings of hope through the positive outlook it cultivates. Maintaining a positive self-esteem through times of trauma will help children better cope with a wide range of emotions and help them persevere through the difficult days ahead.

Here are some ways you can help your children rebuild confidence and feelings of self-worth:

- Always pay attention to what you value about your child and put it into words: "You are so good at taking care of yourself," "Your ideas are important to me," "I admire the way you handled that," "I appreciate your positive outlook," "I can see what a good friend you are."

- Encourage and support friendships that help children feel good about themselves. Help arrange opportunities for your children to spend time with good friends who build them up emotionally and who can be accepting of what they've been through.

- After a trauma it can be empowering for children to put their energy into making a difference in someone else's life or to an important cause. Help children understand that healthy self-esteem is not mere self-absorption.

- Confidence is gained in part by participating in what it is they like to do. Allow children to continue participating in the things they enjoy. You know children are building self-esteem when they are busy having fun and taking pride in what they do or create.

Praise and Reward Your Child

Kids thrive on praise and are motivated by rewards, but since the trauma, your children may not be participating in life like they were before. The stress from trauma can cause children to feel so overwhelmed that they are incapable of performing even the simplest of tasks. When this happens, children lose opportunities to be acknowledged and appreciated.

Now is the time to pay attention to everything your child *is* able to accomplish. You can actually reduce feelings of stress in children and increase feelings of well-being just by giving them ongoing positive reinforcement.

High levels of praise will benefit your child's mood and help them maintain the behaviors you reward. Of course, not all behaviors are ones you wish to reinforce. Some parents find it difficult to praise and reward children who are deeply distressed and acting out in ways the parents don't approve of. Here are some important points to remember about giving praise:

- Lecturing about behavior you don't like may only increase it. Keep your corrections simple and to the point. Your time will be better spent if you praise your child for the qualities and behaviors you respect and admire.

- Don't worry if the qualities and behaviors you want to see more of are sometimes few and far between. Don't give up. The more you notice and admire the qualities you appreciate, the more you'll find your child expressing them.

- Find something to praise and reward every day. Some families enjoy giving daily written praise to one another through a family journal or a note in a lunch box.

- Don't forget to smile.

- Don't forget to give hugs and show your affection.

- Don't forget to say "I love you."

No matter how small or insignificant it might seem, point out the special qualities and abilities you see in your child. Now more than ever, your child needs your encouragement and admiration. Help children understand that the trauma they endured does not have to change all of who they are or wish to be.

The Gift of Feelings

Trusting Feelings

Children don't know what to do with many of the feelings that have engulfed them since the trauma occurred. To resolve the various emotions that will surface, children must learn how to trust what they feel. To do this they will need you to share the following information.

All Feelings Are Normal

Children need to know that everything they feel is normal. It is important for children to understand that whatever reactions they experienced before, during, and after the trauma were common responses for them to have. Encourage children to tell you about the range of reactions they remember experiencing. Let children know that kids who have been through something similar may feel angry, scared, confused, different, and/or lonely. Tell them that all of their feelings are natural.

Listen to Feelings

Children need to be taught how to listen to their feelings. Following a terrifying experience many children are frightened and perplexed by the range of emotions they experience in the moments before, during, and immediately following the trauma. They may no longer want to listen to what they feel. But children need to know that paying attention to their feelings will help them make sense of what happened. Help children understand that even though their feelings were frightening and can't change what already happened, their feelings *can* help protect and guide them in the future.

In the aftermath of trauma, you can help children tune in to how they feel. The best way to help children learn to listen to feelings is to acknowledge the ways you listen to your own feelings.

An example of this is when I denied my daughter the opportunity to spend the night at a new friend's house. She was understandably disappointed. She repeatedly asked, "But why, Mom?! Why can't I?" I didn't have the usual reason, so she felt confused by my decision. She was accustomed to hearing a straightforward answer like, "We have other plans," "We need to get up early," or "Because chores aren't finished." This time I told her that I made the decision to say no because I didn't feel comfortable having her in a home I didn't know enough about. I told her I had learned to trust my feelings, and that even though they weren't always right, I knew my feelings were important to listen to.

I explained to my daughter that I would not risk having her stay somewhere that might not be safe or healthy. I told her my feelings helped me know how to help protect her and keep her safe. I assured her that she could do the same with her feelings. I helped her understand that listening to them could help her make smart choices and decisions. Surprisingly enough, my daughter readily accepted the decision and my explanation. She told me she later realized she felt the same way I did and was actually relieved when I said she couldn't go. Her own developing intuition was in agreement with mine.

When children are faced with their own choices and decisions, encourage them to identify all the thoughts and feelings they have around their options. Listen to them and point out the doubts or ideas you hear that support or deny a certain direction. You might say, "It sounds like you would like to join your friends because you said they are fun to be with, they are really nice, you like them a lot, and you all enjoy skating. Are there any reasons why you wouldn't want to go?" Or, "It sounds like even though you want to go, there are some good reasons why it might be uncomfortable for you to join this group of friends. You said that you've seen them behave in mean ways to other people and that they don't always tell you the truth. You also said you don't like going with kids you don't know very well. That makes good sense to me. It sounds like you can trust your feelings to know whether this is something that will be fun for you to do or not." Remind children that their feelings can't always control situations or predict the future, but that they can be useful guides when facing new experiences and finding ways to help themselves feel better.

Take Their Feelings Seriously

Children's feelings need to be taken seriously. They need to know their feelings will be respected by you. After trauma, children's mixed-up emotions may be hard for them to explain. If they have the ability and words to verbalize what's inside them, they still may be afraid of sounding silly, crazy, or too babyish.

Children can gain inner strength and confidence by hearing your positive responses to whatever they *are* able to share. It is a relief for children to be able to tell you how they feel, but if they judge from your words or behaviors that what they say seems silly or unimportant to you, they will learn to stop sharing. When you don't take your child's feelings seriously, they may interpret this to mean:

- What I have to say doesn't matter.
- What I feel about what happened must be wrong.
- Something is wrong with me.
- Everyone knows what I feel better than I do.
- I don't know what I feel.

In order to help prevent your children from feeling these ways, respond to what they disclose in a calm and serious tone. A minimizing or discounting reaction can cause children to discount their ability for personal insight and it can affect the confidence they have in accurately identifying their feelings.

Understanding Feelings

Help children understand why they feel the way they do. It is important for them to understand that it's normal to have many different feelings for all kinds of reasons. Their understanding of some of the reasons behind their feelings may help explain confusing reactions they've had since the trauma. The more children can understand, the easier they can cope with unwanted or distressing emotions.

Children also need to be assured that feelings can't make bad things happen, that they don't have magic. You can explain that feeling angry at someone, even wishing someone would go away and never come back, cannot make that wish happen. They need to know that telling someone "I wish you would die" cannot kill that person. Explain to your children that everyone has feelings that they later feel sorry about or wish they'd never had.

It is important to help children identify and gain an understanding for the feelings and reactions they personally experienced related to the trauma they had to face.

After my family was impacted by a burglary in our home, my seven-year-old daughter went through a period of intense fear and anger. She was finally able to talk about the reason for her outbursts of rage toward us. She told me she didn't know why she felt the way she did, she just did.

I assured my daughter that once we figured it out, her feelings would help her. We would learn what action to take so that she could feel better. We figured out that she hated her feelings of constant worry and fear but didn't know how to feel better. She got angry and frustrated with herself. That only added to her confusion. She knew we didn't like her taking out her anger on the rest of the family, and she felt ashamed of that, too.

She soon learned that what happened to us was bad, and that she wasn't. She learned this because I took the time to explain it to her. Over a coloring book, on a drive in our car, on a walk to the park, I told her that we can't help feeling the way we do, but we can do a lot of things to change the feelings we don't like. I also reassured her that she was reacting in normal ways to something that had been overwhelming to all of us.

The truth is, the crime made us all angry. As my daughter learned to accept the mixed-up feelings inside her, she started talking about what was making her mad. She was angry that her personal belongings were destroyed and stolen. She was angry that her room didn't feel like her room anymore, instead it felt contaminated. Our home no longer represented safety and comfort for her. She was angry that she didn't feel the way she used to. Every night she worried the "mean people" would come back. She had nightmares about fires and men holding knives to her throat. She was tired of being afraid for her life.

Many children have no idea why they feel the way they do. You can help them learn how to express what they feel, and in time they will probably be able to figure it out. It can help to let them know this.

Once you understand what feelings your child is carrying, you can find ways to help meet special needs and provide comfort. You can do things to help calm fears, ease pain, and rebuild hopes for the future. Children need to be told of your confidence in their ability to heal.

Behaviors Are Feelings Disguised

Changes in behavior are normal reactions to being frightened and upset. Sadness and pain are often expressed through behavior. Many parents are alarmed if a child "acts out" in aggressive and violent ways following a trauma. Acting-out behaviors often communicate anxiety, hurt, fears, and/or underlying depression. It may be the child's attempt to numb him or herself to what happened.

The parents of a ten-year-old boy named Alan came to me expressing concern that he had suddenly started drawing "violent and bizarre" pictures and was engaging in "gun play," which he had not done prior to the shooting he witnessed. I assured his parent's that Alan's play and increased aggressiveness was a normal response to his confusion surrounding the random crime he experienced.

Rather than punish Alan for this behavior, his parents learned to help him play out his feelings in safe ways. They accepted his make-believe world and joined in when invited. His parents helped Alan understand that his play had a purpose. They told him they believed his games were a smart way to help him feel less sad and afraid. They explained that it was normal to try to figure out all the confusing questions and feelings he might have, even while he played and drew pictures. Together Alan and his parents struggled to find answers to the questions they all had about why the traumatic event had happened, how it could happen, why it wasn't stopped in time, why some people didn't survive, and what they would do if it ever happened again. Alan's parents became a powerful resource in their son's recovery. He was no longer alone in his thoughts and feelings.

Five-year-old Jacob was in my office for the first time when he spontaneously started "flying." Every time his parents attempted to tell me about the robbery they endured in their home, he jumped off his chair and "flew" around the room to each piece of furniture he could safely land on. This otherwise shy and withdrawn little boy became animated, loud, and forceful in his behavior. It was the only way he knew how to stop us from talking about what happened and flee the anxiety it produced in him. He continued to "fly away" through out our subsequent sessions whenever he needed to.

Jacob's behavior was an important way he protected himself from feeling overwhelmed. I suspect it was also a way for him to feel he could escape if he found himself in danger again. His illusion of having a magical flying ability soothed his feelings of helplessness and powerlessness. It is important to respect the ingenious ways children take care of themselves.

Difficult Feelings Take Time to Change

You can tell children their feelings may feel mixed up for a while. Explain that some feelings take time to understand and change. In the meantime, you can reassure them by saying:

- It's okay to feel and act differently for a while.

- There are a lot of safe ways that you can take care of yourself.

- Being different can be better when new behaviors help you take care of yourself (like Jacob's need to "fly away" at times).

- It won't always feel this bad.

- You are smart to do things that help you feel better and safer.

- It's okay if you don't feel like you used to.

- You will feel happy again.

- What happened to you has changed you. That's to be expected.

- Life may never feel the same as it did before, but it will get better.

- It will take time to feel better again.

- In time we'll all feel better. Your scary, sad, and angry feelings will go away.

The Recipe for Understanding

"It just takes time" is a familiar phrase. When you tell a child it will take time to make sense of what happened and to feel better again, it can be helpful to illustrate what this means.

You could compare "taking time" to the process of baking bread or cookies. You can explain that first you have ingredients like flour, salt, and baking soda. They don't taste good separately. You mix them together and they begin to taste better. But it's not until you go through the last step of baking that you have a cookie you can eat or a loaf of bread for your sandwich.

Baking is a process much like that of healing. It involves many different steps and ingredients. It takes time to complete. If you rush the process, your cookies and breads won't be done enough to enjoy.

Every recipe requires different amounts of time. In the same way, people require different amounts of time before they are done healing and can begin to feel better again. Understanding feelings is one step in the healing process, but all the steps are important and necessary to complete. Help kids to take the time they need. Help them learn to be patient with themselves by being patient with them.

Expressing Feelings

It is important to tell children they do not have to be alone in their feelings. Help them learn ways to express what they feel with people they love and trust. Regardless of a child's age, parents often find that their child shares many of the same feelings they have. It can be comforting for children to know this.

Because most children do not know how to express their emotions, they will look to you for how to do this. Here is what you can do to show them how:

- Don't hide your own emotions from your children. Instead, let them see the ways you cope with your feelings.

- Don't hide your tears or pretend you are not in pain when you are. Model acceptance for your feelings and reactions.

- Explain to your children how you feel about what happened.

- Tell them why you feel sad and upset.

- Practice sharing how you feel about many situations, not just those involving the trauma.

- Identify all your feelings such as anger, sadness, excitement, happiness, frustration, and loneliness so they will see how to face their own feelings and make sense of them.

What to Say

Help children understand that talking about the feelings they experienced during and after the trauma can help them feel better. Some kids worry that the feelings they have are wrong or bad. It is difficult for them to express feelings to people who might criticize or punish them for feeling the way they do. Children must know there are no wrong feelings. They also need to hear you say it's okay to talk about anything and everything. Here are some things you might say to convey this:

- You don't have to share your thoughts and feelings with everyone, but it's okay to share them with me, or anyone else you trust, when you're ready to talk.

- It's okay to feel sad and cry by yourself. After you've had time to be alone, it will help to talk about how you feel.

- I can listen to whatever it is you would like to tell me about. Your feelings won't worry or frighten me.

- Nothing you feel is wrong. You can tell me anything.

How to Respond

When children begin to express their feelings, you will want to be ready to respond in helpful ways. Here are some suggestions:

- When children are ready to talk, be ready to listen. Stop and be quiet. Give your undivided attention to what your child is saying.

- Repeat what you think you heard them say. Check out if you are understanding what it is they want you to understand. Don't worry about what your perspective is. Just keep listening to theirs.

- Talk more about it. Encourage your child to keep explaining to you how they feel, without judging them.

- Don't ask why they feel the way they do. For now just accept it. They feel the way they do for a reason. You can ask for help in understanding later, but for now, operate from the assumption that there are good reasons for all their feelings.

- Remember to respond rather than react. If you're angry, shocked, blaming, or questioning with judgments or suspicion, your children will not trust you to understand and they may learn to stop talking. Who needs the third degree when you're trying to explain something important inside you? It's counterproductive to healing wounds of the heart.

Using Feelings

Teach children how to use what they feel. Explain that they can use their feelings to help better understand themselves, others, and the world. Following trauma, help children realize that when they trust, understand, and express emotions, they can discover how to use their feelings to help them heal.

What Feelings Can Tell You

Give your child examples of how feelings can show them what they need in order to feel better and take care of themselves:

- When you're *tired,* you know you need to sleep or slow down.

- When you're *lonely,* you need to ask for company and maybe a hug.

- When you're *sad,* you may need to cry, talk, or be alone.

- When you're *angry,* you need to tell someone why. You may need to express to someone why your feelings are hurt.

- When you're *afraid,* you need to find a way to feel safe.

- When you feel *sick,* you may need to go to a doctor or do special things to take care of yourself.

- When you feel *confused,* you need to think and do your best to figure out why.

- When you feel *disappointed,* you learn life does not always give you what you want.

- When you feel *love,* you sometimes need to express it. You can appreciate what and who you love.

- And when you feel *happy,* you learn what you enjoy about life.

Help children learn how to use their feelings through the healing process. If you can help them understand that all of their feelings are valuable parts of themselves, you will have found an important way to assist their recovery.

From the Eyes to the Listening Heart

It only takes seconds to experience a trauma. In a moment or in a glance, a traumatic event can instantly leave it's indelible mark on the heart of a child. One thing is certain: The emotions that follow can take children on an important path in the healing process. It can be the first path on the road to their recovery.

Maria learned to trust, understand, express, and use her feelings in ways that helped empower her recovery. As the key witness at the trial of her baby-sitter's murderer, she told me the pain in her heart would help her tell the truth. She said it would help her remember why it was important to be there showing the judge who the "bad man" was. She told me her anger would help her tell what happened so the man could never kill or hurt anyone again. Her love inspired her to testify because she knew her baby-sitter would be proud of her. Maria clearly wanted to protect other people from the murderer. She said she was afraid but would do it anyway. She would do it for her baby-sitter.

Maria confronted her fears. She never denied the terror she felt of being in the same room with the assailant, but she learned ways to live with the fear. She expressed her pain and openly grieved her loss all along the way. Maria learned that healing happens even in the hurt. Hurting was part of the cure.

In the end, Maria testified beautifully. It was her testimony that resulted in the conviction of the killer. On that day she focused on those of us in the courtroom who loved and supported her. My own tension transformed when she began to speak. I was quickly filled with respect and admiration for this courageous young girl, who just weeks earlier was determined never to speak again. On that day her voice was loud and clear and powerful. She spoke from her heart.   ॐ

2

Healing the Mind

"I can't stop thinking about it."

🖎 *Lisset was sound asleep when her dad rushed to her room at three in the morning. When she heard loud banging and felt the house move, she thought it was another minor earthquake. She wasn't scared. She trusted her dad to protect her. They had survived many small tremors in the ten years they had lived in their home.*

Lisset's slight build made it easy for her dad to lift her, even at the age of eleven. He quickly carried her upstairs and laid her down in a corner behind her parent's bed. She remembers feeling confused for a moment, but was content to be still again and continue on with her dreams. This would be the last night Lisset would sleep so soundly for a long time.

It seemed to Lisset that the whole house began to shake. She was wide awake when the pounding grew louder. She remembers thinking the wall was about to break open and crush her. She had never heard an earthquake sound like this before. When she saw her dad grab a lamp and go downstairs, she realized something was very wrong.

Lisset heard the voice of a stranger outside, screaming obscenities. She realized the ground wasn't causing their home to shake, a "crazy" man was. A flood of questions filled her mind: What was he doing? Would he start shooting? What was wrong with him? Was he alone? Lisset's mother barricaded the door with furniture and ran to help her husband.

The intruder, in a drug-induced rage, made no secret of his intentions. He threatened to kill everyone inside once he got in. Clinging to a pillow, Lisset remained huddled alone in the dark corner of her parent's room. She began to shake and cry uncontrollably. Lisset heard her parents on the phone to the police. Over and over again she heard them scream, "He's in the house! He's in the house! He's inside the house now!" They were yelling in a way she had never heard before. Lisset thought her parents were being killed.

The assailant seriously injured two police officers before he could be subdued. Lisset's parents narrowly escaped harm by dodging his violent attempts to assault them. They suffered only minor cuts caused by broken glass, but the emotional assault left the family with permanent scars.

Lisset never saw the assailant nor witnessed the trauma visually, but what she heard was imprinted in her memory forever. She saw pictures in her mind from what she heard, and like a movie in her head, they played over and over again. Lisset was consumed by fear during the day and terrorized by dreams at night. The trauma had left her incapacitated. The only time she left her bedroom was to see that all the locks in the house remained secure. Lisset refused to go to school. She could not bear to be separated from her parents. She could not stop thinking about the need to check every lock in the house.

Lisset asked her parents for help. She asked them to find her someone who could make her forget what happened.

When I met Lisset, she walked timidly into my office. She sat down nervously, her hands and mouth trembling. She chose to have her parents with her the first time she came to see me. I told her she could stay with them as long as she needed to and to let me know when she was ready to be without them in my office.

I gave Lisset and her parents permission to share what they wanted to about that night. I told them it was important to go at their own pace. I let them know I would not expect them to describe anything they didn't feel ready to and asked them to help me understand what that night had been like for each of them. Lisset looked anxiously to her mom to begin. As her mom described what happened in general terms, they both began to cry.

Lisset told me she wanted to come to counseling to find out what to do with her "bad and scary thoughts." She said she didn't like talking about what happened because she already felt too scared *from thinking about it all the time. She said, "I can't stop thinking about it. I must be going crazy! I can't leave my room because when I do, I have to keep checking the locks, even when I know I already did. All day long I have a movie of it in my brain! Can't you just give me a pill or something to make me forget it?"*

Lisset had a wound so deep it filled her mind with fear. In the weeks ahead, I learned just how powerful a medicine feeling safe again was to her recovery. The healing process could not continue without it.   ◈

Trauma Leaves Painful Memories

Trauma affects thoughts as well as feelings. A wide range of memories can complicate the healing process and prolong the most frightening aspects of a child's experience. When this happens, there is no peace of mind. It is important to help children learn how to live with the memory of what happened so it won't interfere with their continued development. When distressing thoughts can be shared, they can be put to rest. Children may tell you what they're thinking about in many different ways.

Thoughts That Won't Stop

Following trauma, some children will describe what they experienced over and over again. They will talk to anyone who will listen. There may be a sense of urgency in their voice as they continually retell the story of what happened. Children become anxious when life doesn't make sense to them.

Repetitious questions and discussions happen when children have heard information they don't understand or have experienced something they can't make sense of. Understanding takes time. Children may need to hear the same answers many times before they're able to "get" it.

The details or questions that children repeatedly bring up to you may cause you to experience personal feelings of helplessness. You can't change what happened, but you can help children come to terms with their distress. Allowing them to freely express what's on their minds can help. As difficult or tiring as it can be to hear, it is important to listen with a supportive and open attitude. It is helpful when children can express everything that's on their minds to a caring adult. The more the story is told, the less troubling the thoughts are to live with.

A mother expressed concern to me about her four-year-old daughter, Lindsay. Ever since her grandmother was attacked and killed, her daughter asked questions and wanted details about the crime constantly. The mother, in distress herself, found her daughter's need to talk about the murder unbearable. It was important for her to deal with her own reactions to the trauma before she could cope effectively with her daughter.

Unexpected Disclosures

Not all children want to talk repeatedly about what happened to them. Instead, they might share at unexpected times and in unexpected ways. You may be surprised when your child suddenly discloses something he or she has been concerned about or fearful of This often happens when you least expect it.

In a checkout line at the grocery store, Lisset told her mom that since the break-in, she thought she saw a man with a butcher knife at her bedroom window every night.

I also counseled Jeremy, a five-year-old boy whose room had been torn apart during a burglary. Just as he was about to close the car door as his mother dropped him off for school one morning, he leaned in and said, "The bad guys are up in the attic at night waiting to kill me."

In both cases, the parents learned valuable information about their child's deepest fears. With this new information they learned how to respond, comfort, and reassure their children in different ways. This increased their child's ability to cope. Listening to children's fears will help relieve the lonely burden they often carry in silence, as well as enable you to respond in helpful ways.

Children Need to Speak Their Minds

It's important for children to put their thoughts outside of themselves, especially if they are experiencing a constant replay of memories, so these memories can begin to subside. It's important not only to know what they were feeling, but also what they were thinking about before, during, and after the traumatic event. This information, from children's own unique perspective, will help you understand their deepest fears and worries. It will also allow distressing memories to be purged. The relief most children experience when this happens cannot be underestimated.

The No-Talk Rule

Sometimes families have spoken or unspoken "rules" for not talking about the event or certain details involving the trauma. Never urge your child to "forget about it." Discussion of the event should be supported and encouraged if your child wants to discuss it (Pynoos and Eth 1985c; Figley 1988). It's best not to limit children's discussion by prohibiting them from saying or expressing certain aspects of the experience they went through (Bowlby 1980). Questions concerning who, what, where, why, and how can help children get the details out when they want to talk. Be willing to hear everything as many times as it needs to be said.

Helping Children Tell the Story

It's important to help children feel free to speak their minds and to voluntarily tell you about their experiences of what happened. Never force or pressure them to tell you anything they are not yet willing to verbalize. Once they feel safe and comfortable, they may want to share with you what they went through. Here is a list of what you can say to support children who are ready to tell you their story:

- It's often helpful to talk about what happened.

- Talking about what happened can help you let go of painful thoughts and memories.

- Draw a picture of what's in your mind. Write a story about what's in your mind.

- Thoughts cannot make bad things happen or prevent them from happening.

- I can handle whatever you would like to tell me about. Your thoughts don't scare or worry me.

- Anything you think about is normal for what you have been through.

- How do you imagine you might think about this in the future (e.g., in one week; three months; five years; when you're a grown-up)?

- Having frightening thoughts does not mean you are going crazy. What happened was crazy, you are not.

- The trauma is over. You have survived the pain it caused, and with time you will survive the memory, too.

- It's important to talk about what you're going through and what you've been through when you are ready.

- What is your understanding of what happened?

- What do you know about it?

- What do you want to know?

- What do you wonder about it?

- Where were you when it happened?

- What were you doing?

- How did you hear about it?

- Who was involved? Who else was there?

- What did you think about when it happened?

- What did you say to yourself?

- What do you remember seeing, hearing, smelling, touching, and/or tasting?

- What most concerned you?

- What's your most painful moment or memory?

- What was your first reaction?

- What's not being talked about?

- Are other people right or wrong about what they're saying happened?

- What was handled well?

- Who was helpful and why?

- All of your thoughts before, during, and after the event are normal.

When Children Don't Confide

Sometimes children need someone other than their parents or family to confide in. Children may find it more stressful to experience their parents' reactions than to keep their thoughts to themselves.

They may want to protect you from what they experienced for many reasons. They may worry that their reactions and fears will be too frightening for loved ones to deal with, or they may fear that their family's questions and concerns will never stop. Children may worry that their family will want to talk about what happened, even when they don't.

If your child refuses to talk, never force the issue. It's not always easy to verbalize thoughts and memories, even when children want to. Continue to encourage them by communicating your own belief that sharing with someone when they are ready can be helpful.

Children often require outside support in order to talk freely about their experience. Chapter 5 will help you sort through the decision of seeking professional help for your child.

Children Will Ask What They Need to Know

After a tragedy, the need for understanding is real. Children may want more information in their attempt to resolve their questions and confusion. It is difficult for children to heal when they are denied information that can help them.

Children may surprise you with questions you don't feel prepared to answer. Let them know you're glad they've asked anyway. Acknowledge questions and information about the trauma honestly and in a calm, serious, and nondramatic way. Children need enough information to understand what happened without becoming overwhelmed.

The mother of a four-year-old girl learned to answer her daughter's questions and concerns about her grandmother's murder by saying, "Yes, it's true. Your grandmother was hurt so badly that she couldn't get better. When someone dies, they cannot come back." When she asked why her mother was crying, her mother answered, "I feel sad when I talk about what happened, because I miss her." To her daughter's questions about why it happened she replied, "Most people are very good, but the man who hurt grandma was not." And to her daughter's questions about how the man killed her grandmother she explained, "The man hurt grandma with a knife."

To resolve troubling thoughts and memories children may seek more information about what happened from outside sources, especially if they can't find answers from you. They may look to friends, television shows, newspaper reports, or radio programs to find out more. It's important for children to receive accurate information, but it's also important not to expose them to sources that can traumatize them further. They may hear inaccurate information or hear more than they can handle.

Guidelines for Sharing Information

In order to help your children come to terms with what happened, let them understand what they need to know in a loving and protective manner. Here are some suggestions for how to do this:

- Answer all questions.

- Tell the truth.

- When there are no answers, be honest about that, too.

- Keep answers simple and direct.

- Clarify misinformation.

- Give accurate facts and details surrounding the event to help children integrate their memories.

- Be as factual as possible without providing graphic details. This avoids overstimulating a child's imagination.

- Don't lie to protect your child. Offering inaccurate information can slow down the recovery process as well as affect their trust in you.

- Don't expect children to comprehend the same information adults receive. Make explanations easy for them to understand.

- Make it your job to be a buffer for your children when you can. Protect them from being exposed to what is unnecessary to see or hear. Broadcast news, movies, television shows, and even newspapers can offer graphic pictures and images that may increase their anxiety.

- Remember that the more children understand, the less fearful they will be.

Fear and Safety

Following trauma, the two most common issues on a child's mind are fear and safety. Children who were direct witnesses to crime usually fear retaliation and having to testify in court. Those who lived close to where the trauma happened or felt personally threatened are likely to feel more vulnerable. However, kids who were further removed from the incident may be no less affected, as they often think, "If it can happen to them, it can happen to me."

Children need to know that it's normal to feel frightened and upset by some of their thoughts and ideas. They also need to know that you will help them cope with their fears and find ways to feel safe and protected again.

Fears of death and further trauma preoccupy many children. They may be perplexed because they feel scared at times and places that used to feel safe to them, such as school, church, or a store. Many children I have worked with have expressed the fear that their disturbing thoughts would interfere with their life forever.

Lisset felt "different" about life after the break-in. She hadn't worried about death before the trauma. She told me once, "Death can hit you anywhere, nothing is safe." She expressed her fears about nuclear war, drive-by shootings, and a person on the street who had frightened her. She worried about religious persecution since a nearby temple had been bombed the previous week. Lisset said she was "jumpy" every time she heard a loud voice. Even people she could see worried her when they yelled.

One evening Lisset's father accidentally dropped a jar of mayonnaise on the kitchen floor and yelled at himself out of frustration. Lisset told me she felt her heart stop. She immediately thought, "My daddy's getting killed!"

In another incident, the soccer coach at Lisset's school startled her during a game. He yelled at the team in an un- expected outburst and she became so shaken that she went to the bathroom and cried inside the bathroom stall. Lisset told me no one else seemed to mind his yelling. She said she felt she did not "belong" in her group of friends anymore. She felt alienated and alone. She experienced life as dangerous and unpredictable. Lisset said what happened had changed her forever. She believed she would never be the same.

In time, with counseling, Lisset learned ways to cope with her frightening thoughts and ideas. She learned relaxation exercises, which she practiced in the day and used at night. She began writing her "scary thoughts" in a book that she could lock away afterwards. She refused to use her diary because she said she didn't want to look back and remember this experience when she was older.

Lisset accepted the fact that I couldn't give her pills to make her forget what had happened, but she still hoped I had counseling techniques that would "erase" the memory. When I told her I preferred to help her learn how to live with the memory, Lisset looked disappointed. I assured her she could remember the trauma in the future without becoming overwhelmed by it. I told her it did not have to affect how she chose to live the rest of her life and assured her she would be able to walk through life again without thinking danger lurked around every corner.   ✑

How to Help Conquer Fears

When children feel frightened by thoughts, images, and ideas that are scary or worrisome, help them conquer their fears by using the following suggestions:

- Ask, "What can I do to help?" or "What would help you the most right now?"

- Increase physical contact and comforting, but remember that all the comfort in the world can't erase what happened.

- Acknowledge your children's fears and remind them that everyone has fearful thoughts.

- Reassure children by telling them, "We will work through your fearful thoughts together."

- Lower your expectations of your child's day-to-day performance and activities.

- Don't be afraid to hear your child's thoughts.

- Be present when you're with your child.

- Help children understand that even though their thoughts may seem confusing, they have good reasons for thinking the way they do.

- Tell your child it is normal to think differently after something so different happens.

- Offer ways to cope when you can.

- Practice relaxation techniques together (see Resources for book and tapes on relaxation skills).

- Explain that thoughts and feelings do eventually become less frightening once they are fully expressed.

- Indulge special needs for a time so that a sense of security may be reconstructed.

- Sometimes you must look deeper to discover the source of your child's fears. Seek a professional's help if you need more assistance. You and your child may benefit from learning new ways to cope with fear and anxiety. Therapists can teach effective ways to desensitize children from chronic fears or phobias.

- Let your child need you.

The What-ifs, Should-haves, and If-onlys

Like adults, some children will express deep regret at not having been able to change the course of events they experienced. They may ask themselves and others, "What if I would have gone here instead of there?" or "I should have done this instead of that," or "If only I had known, I could've done something different." These "what-ifs" and "shoulds" are an attempt to resolve some of their fears. Children might hope to prevent another similar experience by determining what their alternatives were or what they "should" have done differently. By retracing their steps they also create a distraction from what really happened. It's an important way the mind tries to sift through difficult memories and change or dispose of them.

A girl who had been harassed by school bullies asked herself repeatedly, "What if I would've walked the way I usually do? Maybe this would've never happened," or "If only I would have stayed home from school today!", "What if I could've looked up sooner to see them walking toward me," "I should have screamed instead of froze," and "I should have been able to handle it."

Children need to know that questioning their choices and actions is a natural step in the process of coming to terms with a harrowing experience. Eventually, memories are integrated and the mind can no longer be fooled. Children often come to a point when they realize that all of the analyzing and retracing of steps they could ever do won't change what really happened.

It's been said that in hindsight everyone has perfect vision. It is important to remind children that there are no crystal balls to see into the future or help them avoid consequences for every move and step they take in the world. Explain that part of life is not knowing what's ahead, and a small part of life is not being able to prevent or change what comes your way.

What If It Happens Again?

One of the greatest fears children have about trauma is wondering if it will happen again. This is an important question that needs to be acknowledged and addressed honestly. It is a question adults are almost always asked.

Some parents would like to respond to this question by saying, "You don't have to worry about that," "It will never happen again," or "It could never happen again." But what if it could? And what if it does? It is better to discuss the possibility than to mislead a child.

Parents can be honest without catastrophizing or instilling chronic fear and anxiety in children. Here are some ways to answer the question "What if it happens again?" honestly:

- You're right. It could happen again even though it probably won't.

- We can talk about what we would do if it happened again.

- We can't know everything that will happen in life, but we can be prepared for most things that happen.

- You're safe now and it's not likely that you'll ever have to go through this again.

- There are a lot of things we can do to help you stay safe.

- I will continue to do everything in my power to protect you.

Children need to be assured that you will do everything possible to help them stay safe. Following the burglary in our home, we decided to spend the insurance money we received on an alarm system. Within two days of receiving the settlement check, our little house was equipped like San Quentin. "So what," we decided. We could feel safe again. The peace of mind it helped restore was worth it.

Lisset's parents took steps to increase their feelings of safety, too. They began by having the police inspect their home and offer suggestions for improvements. They were able to install additional locks and improve existing ones. A security alarm system and watch dog were also helpful additions.

Regaining Power and Control

When the world goes "crazy," as it does during a traumatic event, children lose their sense of power and control over life. Their sense of security has been stolen. How do you help them get it back?

I tell families they will get their bearings and their sense of security back slowly, day by day, as they return to normalcy, to routines, to the ordinary schedules of their lives. In the meantime, let children choose to take the steps they need to take in order to feel safe again.

🙠 *Lisset chose to sleep with her closet door open with a lamp on inside it. She rearranged her furniture so that it barricaded the window. She used a night light on the other side of her room and listened to soft music to try to help her relax. Every day she decided how many times she would check and recheck the locks in their home. Lisset decided when her parents could leave her alone again in the house.*

In an attempt to help her control the increasing obsession she had with the house locks, I gave Lisset the homework assignment of checking the locks twice as much as she had been doing. I asked her to keep a log of the number of times she was able to increase her "checking." I explained to Lisset that her behavior served an important purpose. I understood from her that she still did not feel safe enough in her home. Her fears were grounded in reality. They were based on what had really happened. It was normal and healthy to desire safety.

I told Lisset I believed that her constant checking of locks was a good idea. She and her family deserved to know they were safe. However, I told her she needed to do it more because it wasn't working enough yet. Lisset laughed at me and thought I was joking. She was delighted to learn that I was serious. The following week she explained how difficult it was to continue checking the locks as much as I had instructed her to. She told me that in fact she'd stopped. And she was relieved. It had grown too tiring for her, and she knew she could check the locks whenever she needed to. She told me she knew it was her decision now. She was no longer controlled by the thought that doors and windows might be unlocked. She trusted herself to know she was accurate the first time she checked.

Lisset also learned to take power and control over her nightmares. She began a journal of her dreams and learned to rewrite them with different endings. She learned to finish her dreams by taking power and control in them. She became the hero, with strength and courage. She wrote about the ways her new home successfully protected her family. Lisset's nightmares became less disturbing as they took on the endings she had created. She began to sleep more restfully again. 🙠

What You Can Do

Just as children need to be given choices about when and what they will share about their experience, part of your job as a loving parent is to help them regain a sense of power and control. Here's how to help:

- Give your child plenty of choices. Give options in day-to-day decision making whenever possible (e.g., what they eat, wear, or do that day).

- Respect your child's opinions and suggestions.

- Respect the choices your child makes.

- Acknowledge to yourself and your child that there are no right or wrong thoughts or ways to think following a traumatic life event.

- Trust what your children say they need (i.e., to check the locks, keep the light on, have people near them, be given time alone).

Change Can Be Positive

Eventually Lisset's family moved to a new home. Her parents wondered if moving was really "running away." They were concerned that moving might be counterproductive to their family's recovery. I told them I believed some fears can be faced, while other fears inspire positive changes. Most importantly, children and their families need to do whatever they can to feel safe. Changing environments and beginning anew can be an excellent choice when it is understood by everyone. Change can be symbolic of taking back power and control.

School Life

Pain can emerge at any point. For some kids, reactions may appear in the distant future. Older children may respond in the same ways they see their peers behaving, and so they may initially seem unmoved, apathetic, or uncaring. They may feel embarrassment and fear about exposing true feelings. Reactions can then become problematic later on, often showing up in the form of difficulties in school.

Schools that provide continual screening and follow-up for all children impacted by a traumatic event provide a significant service. As a parent, it will be helpful to be aware of any delayed reactions your child might show at school so that you can intervene and be supportive if and when it happens.

Trauma Impacts Learning

Children cannot learn when they're not relaxed. Some children are in a constant state of anxiety following a trauma. Depression and lack of sleep are also factors that interfere with learning.

Some children may appear as if they are in another world. It is common for them to experience difficulties in memory and concentration. In school, they may appear distracted, less attentive, and preoccupied. A common complaint I have heard from children whose school work and grades suffered after witnessing trauma was that they had trouble trying to make "scary thoughts" and "pictures in their mind" stop. It distracted them from their daily tasks and routines.

Intrusive thoughts and images—sudden mental pictures or memories of what happened or what is feared—plague many children. Even though one nine-year-old girl I worked with had never seen a gun or witnessed a shooting, she described seeing machine guns at her window every night after seeing a neighbor physically assaulted. Her overwhelming fear and insecurity in the world had transferred itself to the threat of war and personal danger.

When Lisset was able to share her experience of the break-in with me, she described seeing pictures in her mind that "flashed on like a light." She told me she saw her dad screaming into the phone. She saw the dark corner of the room she was hiding in. She saw the wall caving in and crushing her. She saw her mom's face as she struggled to push furniture into a protective barricade for her. She saw a man striking her parents to the ground. She saw her mom crying in pain. Lisset said, "I can see it all the time, even when I try not to. It ruins everything. I can't concentrate on anything at school. I can't do anything but try to make it stop." Lisset learned that the more she shared the images with me, the easier they were to contain. She learned to use bright red stop signs in her mind when she became distressed by her thinking. When Lisset learned to accept all of her thoughts and feelings, and stopped avoiding them, they lost their power. It no longer became a fierce battle to stop them or try to prevent them from happening.

Worry about Loved Ones

It is difficult for most kids to be away from loved ones following a tragedy. It may be especially hard for children to be at school and separated from those they care about. Like Lisset, most kids will have periods of time where they are preoccupied with worry about loved ones and find themselves struggling to concentrate and listen in class.

Lisset told me she worried that the man who broke into their house would come back and kill her mom and dad while she was at school. Staying home and close to them gave her greater security. Children's fear may be intensified by separation. Being physically close to loved ones reassures them that they are safe and the trauma is not happening again. For a period of two weeks, Lisset found it helpful to call home on her lunch and recess breaks. Her teacher facilitated this plan, which proved to be very helpful. Lisset could then sit in class and breathe a little easier.

Classroom Behaviors

Some children react differently and find comfort from being in school. They may want to work harder because it enables them to forget about what happened. Still others may become disruptive and restless and experience difficulties controlling their own behaviors. Consequently, it is not unusual for school performance to be impaired for a time.

It will be helpful if your child's teacher can adjust for these predictable effects. It is not realistic to expect traumatized children to maintain their usual performance. It is appropriate and helpful for teachers to accommodate your child's symptoms unless they are unsafe or interfering with other students' learning. Placing pressure on a child to improve performance, giving negative consequences, and disciplining are likely to exacerbate symptoms. Be sure you know what's happening in your child's life at school.

Working with Your Child's Teacher

Parents and teachers can brainstorm strategies together that will make school life easier. Being an advocate for your child is especially important at this time.

To help your child's readjustment to school, stay in close communication with teachers and other personnel who have contact with your child. Most will welcome the ideas and knowledge you have about your child. The information you share can assist teachers in ways that will help them support your child and ensure their continued success.

The following suggestions are actions you can take to help children gain the necessary help and support they will need at school:

- As soon as possible after an event call the school guidance counselor to inform the principal and teacher about the trauma that impacted your children and the effects it has had on them.

- Share any special needs or concerns you have.

- Depending on the type of trauma your children have suffered, let the teacher know if they're sensitive to loud bells, sirens, or crowds, and help the teacher prepare to offer support to your children at those times.

- Children may have trouble keeping food down and should not be forced to eat. Let appropriate school personnel know in case it is a lunchtime policy to finish all food.

- Children may feel anxious about playing games on the playground that involve playing "dead." Ask that school personnel be sensitive to this and redirect play when possible. Ask if there are limits set around inappropriate kinds of play on the playground as well as in the classroom and, if so, what "inappropriate play" includes.

- Any number of factors could trigger feelings of fear. Help your child's teacher to be aware of as many of them as you know so that he or she can respond reassuringly if your child experiences difficulties.

- Help and encourage your child's teacher to consult regularly with everyone involved in your child's life. If your child is seeing a counselor, give your child's teacher permission verbally and in writing to consult with the counselor and vice versa.

- Help your child's teacher understand the importance of rebuilding a sense of security at school. A skillful and sensitive teacher will help maintain a structure and routine the student is comfortable with. Any specific suggestions or ideas you can share about how to do this will be invaluable.

Homework and Grades

Let teachers know you approve of allowing your children the opportunity to complete work at their own pace. You can help rebuild confidence by reassuring children that in time they will be able to do their best work again. In the meantime, ask that they be given permission to do only what they're able to.

It is not uncommon for an otherwise average to outstanding student to drop grades down to the failing point. Teachers need to know that *symptoms prevent kids from performing at their usual level* and sometimes accommodating special needs works in everyone's best interest. You might suggest that your children be encouraged to take control of homework by making their own decisions about it for a while. Ask that they be allowed to determine what they can and cannot realistically accomplish. For example, a student may feel confident about completing a two-page report but not ten pages, or ten math problems instead of twenty.

Some teachers may worry that their students will fall too far behind or take advantage of the "break" this gives them. But you can remind them that a traumatized student who is experiencing difficulties with school work is already falling behind. To continue to pile on more assignments will only overwhelm and slow them down further. You might want to encourage your child's school to reconsider some policies when trauma has interfered with school performance. For example, middle school and older students may benefit from a pass / no pass agreement rather than letter grades.

Teachers can help your children gradually return to their level of functioning by working with them in an empowering way that lets them decide when and how much they can get done. Requirements don't have to change, but you can suggest that the timetable and methods to satisfy assignments can.

Feeling Different

Suffering from a traumatic event that most people never experience or witnessing something no one else has may cause children to feel "branded" or different.

Children may complain that their friends ignore them or leave them out of games and activities on purpose. Usually it helps to explain to children that trauma makes everyone feel afraid. Tell children that people may ignore them because they are really afraid of what happened. They may not know what to say or how to act around them, knowing they've been through something so tragic. Reassure your child that they are not to blame, and that this situation is temporary.

If sarcastic remarks, name calling, or teasing are a problem, help your child decide on the best course of action to take. Let your child know that they don't have to tolerate the disrespect of others, though they shouldn't retaliate by being disrespectful as a way to stop it. Practice assertive responses with them and help identify an adult they can seek out who can intervene if necessary.

When Rumors Hurt

Stories about the trauma your child and family has suffered can quickly circulate. Sometimes more lies than facts are spread among classmates, neighbors, or community groups you have contact with. Here are some ways you can help your children cope with hurtful gossip:

- Help your child understand that rumors are spread by children and adults who often have little else to do.

- Explain that resorting to gossip that wounds and offends is cruel, insensitive, and wrong. It does violence against a person's character. They have a right to feel hurt by it.

- Tell your children that some people spread untrue stories because they think it's fun and they like the attention it gives them.

- Explain that most people who gossip don't know or think about how hurtful their actions are to those they spread rumors about.

- Make sure they understand that they can't control rumors, but they can control the way they respond to them.

- Encourage them to ignore, correct, or confront rumors to handle malicious talk.

- Ask that they don't try to teach the people spreading stories a lesson by starting their own rumors about them; retaliation won't stop what's happening, but it will make an even bigger problem.

- Recommend that they reconsider being friends with someone who is unwilling to respond respectfully to their feelings.

- Suggest that they surround themselves with people who like, love, believe in, and support them.

- Ask that they don't spend time with people or "friends" who put your children down or cause them to feel self-doubt or sadness.

- Recommend that they pick friends who like your children for who they are, no matter what they've been through.

If the Media Calls

The public's right to information usually overrides your family's right to privacy. Homicide, suicide, and violent crime make headlines. The media can intrude at the very times you need your privacy the most. They may even show up at your child's school or other places where you believed you would be left alone. Sometimes information can be made public without concern for the impact it may have on your family.

If you are contacted by the media, you might feel challenged. Their questions could feel inappropriate or insensitive. There are many reporters who are respectful and fair, but you may not know if you have one of them interviewing you. Be prepared. Coach your children to go to a trusted grown-up if they are approached. Keep the following in mind:

- You have the right to refuse to talk to the media.

- You can choose to give a simple one or two sentence statement or write it down and hand it to the press.

- Here's an example of what you might say: "We are experiencing a great deal of trauma from this tragedy and must refrain from public comment. Please honor our request by respecting the needs of our children and family."

- If there is a legal case involved, it is always a good idea to contact your attorney before speaking to the media.

- In case the media shows up at school, be sure staff members understand the steps you wish them to take to protect your child from such intrusions.

- Be sure that anyone seeking information from your child will be sensitive and skilled. Nurses, doctors, police officers, and other helping professionals *usually* have special training designed to meet the special needs of children. A neighbor or media person, on the other hand, may have none. Protect your child from those who may be well intentioned but lack tact. Information could be shared that your child was not aware of yet. They may unintentionally traumatize your child further.

School Violence

Children and their parents have cause for concern regarding the increasing climate of violence in schools. It is important to pay attention and take responsibility for your child's school environment. Every school can and should work toward creating an atmosphere free from harassment, bullying, and violence. Children cannot learn in an intimidating climate.

How Adults Can Help

All children, staff, and visitors need to feel safe at school. There are many ways parents and volunteers can contribute to the creation of a safe and respectful environment. Here are some things you can do:

- Be involved at your child's school at all grade levels.

- Help develop a tolerance for frustration by saying no to your child when it's in their best interest. Saying no to your child at an early age will help them learn how to cope with feelings of anger, frustration, and disappointment. Frustrations with school life can be easier to accept and accommodate when kids have had practice at home.

- Encourage your child to remain active and participate in activities that provide positive adult role models in peer activities such as music, sports, and clubs.

- Help children become critical thinkers. Talk about violence in the media and the message it sends. Talk about the consequences of violent acts and point out what might be unrealistic about them. Teach children to identify harmful as well as positive messages in the media.

- Trust your intuition. If you are concerned about your child, seek help and be persistent about it.

- Teach children to recognize the signs and symptoms of students who may be in distress. Identify the adult(s) they should go to with any concerns.

- Consider ways you can be a presence in your child's schools. Act as a mentor, guide, mediator, and/or model for children, emphasizing respectful relationships. Show that fighting and all forms of physical and verbal aggression will not be tolerated or accepted. A child's sense of security is increased by seeing adults function in this capacity for them.

- Some schools train students to assist and support fellow classmates in crisis. "Peer group helpers" can be very effective and can increase a sense of community among students at school.

- Encourage your school to set an important example and adopt or improve on a warm and welcoming "customer service" approach toward all children.

Learning to Live with the Memory

Children can grow strong in spite of trauma, but strength and courage can only be discovered when children feel safe again. The healing process does not continue without it. Children need to be reassured that you will do whatever you can to help them feel safe. It is only through sharing the thoughts and memories that haunt them that children find peace of mind again. Acceptance comes from remembering, not forgetting. Learning to live with traumatic memories is not unlike the process of healing a physical wound.

I explained to Lisset that healing from trauma was like healing from an appendicitis attack. It would never be okay that it happened. It would always be a part of her memory. And it was very painful. Surgery was even required to fix it. The discomfort and pain following surgery was severe. Some days were worse than others. But gradually as the wound continued to heal, it would become easier to do the things she used to. Physically, she would begin to feel like her old self again. Over time, the scar that remained would remind her of that awful day when she had suffered so. And with more time the scar she had now grown accustomed to seeing would become a part of herself. When she looked at it she would even forget the pain it stood for. She would adjust to the scar and realize that she had survived the experience. Her scar could be proof of how well she survived and of her own body's amazing ability to heal itself.

I continued to give Lisset hope. I shared continuously my belief that she would feel whole again and helped her believe in and look forward to that day.

In her last session, Lisset said she realized she was never "crazy." She thanked me for giving her the strength and courage to get over her fears. I explained to Lisset that I hadn't given her anything and told her I simply helped her find what was inside herself all along. Lisset smiled and said, "I never knew I had so much strength and courage in me already! It makes me feel good because I know now that it's there to use again whenever I need to."

3

Healing the Body

"I get weak and dizzy, and I feel like I'm going to die."

✍ *Stacy and her best friend's family were lucky to be alive. They never imagined that going out to eat would be a life-threatening and life-altering experience. They would never eat out again without remembering the Saturday morning when they were victims of a one-man shooting spree.*

The family had just paid for breakfast and were about to leave. As they approached the front doors, a gunman behind them open fired on customers sitting at the booths and tables. The adults with Stacy instinctively shielded her and the two other children with them. She was pushed out the door and onto the ground behind bushes. Shots shattered the windows above them and people stood stunned in the parking lot. Bystanders reported hearing the cries of babies and the screams of injured people inside. One person was killed and five were critically wounded by the time the crime spree ended. Two hours later Stacy was reunited with her parents, who cried when they saw her.

For the next three months, Stacy experienced dizziness and fainting spells. It grew increasingly worse, and no one understood why. At first they didn't believe it could be related to the crime she witnessed. All of Stacy's friends and family talked about how fortunate she had been not to be injured. They also expressed relief that she didn't remember much.

Stacy was an active eleven-year-old before she witnessed the shooting. Now, the fear of fainting prevented her from participating with friends in soccer, slumber parties, and the summer camp she had always looked forward to attending. Life felt too risky even for bike riding in front of her home. Stacy lacked energy and enthusiasm. She appeared disinterested and detached from what she was doing most of the time. Doctors recommended counseling for Stacy to help her with what they believed were stress-related symptoms. She was referred to my office for help.

In the first few weeks of counseling, I asked Stacy to keep a written list of her symptoms of dizziness and a log of dates and times they occurred. She described for me what she was doing before and during the spells, where she was, when it started and ended, and who was around each time it happened. No patterns emerged. The incidents seemed to be unrelated to anything happening around her. Stacy told me, "It happens everywhere. I get weak and dizzy and I feel like I'm going to die." Stacy could begin to feel dizzy and light-headed at home watching television, shopping with her mother, driving in the car, or standing in an elevator. It didn't seem to matter where it happened or who she was with. Most of the time she would end up fainting.

Together, Stacy and I began exploring all that she remembered of the trauma. She talked openly and directly about the fact that she remembered seeing and hearing very little of what actually took place. Stacy did remember the smell of dirt and juniper bushes. She was also able to tell me about some of her thoughts during the incident. She remembered wishing she had stayed home with her parents. She wondered what they were doing while she was being "shot at." Stacy remembered little else of that morning except the feeling of how much she wanted her parents.

Stacy had a wound so deep, her body became ill. In the weeks ahead, I learned what a powerful medicine remembering could be. It would provide the understanding of the physical symptom interfering with Stacy's life and ultimately provide the cure.

When Trauma Has Physical Effects

Trauma can impact the physical health and well-being of children. Physical sensations as well as emotional reactions can become problematic in the aftermath of trauma. Your child's doctor should always be consulted to determine whether symptoms are stress related or not.

Stress from trauma can take a toll on the body. Not eating, or feeling weak, exhausted, anxious, and fearful, can wear you down physically. The long-term effects stress can have on every system in the body is well documented. It is important to help children manage the stress they feel in order to minimize the impact on their physical health.

Physical Memories

Children feel what they've seen. Even when they haven't literally "seen" an event, they may have attached pictures or a physical memory to it. Whatever they saw, heard, smelled, touched, tasted, or remember—from the moment they knew something was wrong until the trauma was over—is likely to be imprinted somewhere deep inside them.

Lack of sleep, stomachaches, nervousness, and headaches are common complaints. These symptoms and others like them may come out of the sense of helplessness from having to watch or listen to the sights and sounds surrounding a traumatic event. The same symptoms of distress may occur for a child who had no direct contact with the experience themselves but knew or even heard of someone who did.

Physical symptoms may or may not be directly related to the actual event your child was exposed to. One child I worked with said her stomach hurt whenever her mother left her. She remembered her stomach being "in knots" when she saw her mother assaulted, and she subsequently developed stomachaches whenever she was separated from her mother. Another child was unable to reestablish regular sleep patterns in the months following a gang shooting she witnessed. Nightmares and bed-wetting interrupted her sleep throughout the night. The lack of sleep caused severe fatigue and unrelenting headaches through the day. All of these symptoms are examples of how anxiety may include physical symptoms with no physical cause.

A six-year-old girl I worked with began stuttering whenever she spoke about the fatal car accident she witnessed. She robotically repeated her sentences, stuttering through the same words again and again. When she learned to talk to me about the trauma through art and puppet play, the stuttering stopped and did not return.

It's common for children who've been exposed to trauma to experience nightmares, be easily startled and jumpy, and feel apprehensive and overly cautious. Children who are usually calm may appear agitated, and active children may become lethargic. Fatigue, increased colds or flu, and changes in appetite or eating habits are also common.

Very young children do not have the capability of remembering an event in their mind, but they may hold on to a physical memory of the tragedy. Joshua was an eighteen-month-old toddler who showed many new behaviors after witnessing a violent crime resulting in his aunt's death. He began crying in a high-pitched scream and was more tearful in general. He began climbing out of his crib at all hours of the night to find his mother. He was successful in making his way out even when his mother went to greater lengths to keep him in his crib. Knowing how important increased physical contact is to children of any age following a trauma, I asked Joshua's mother to hold him a minimum of three times a day in a rocking chair for at least twenty minutes each time. The following week Joshua was sleeping through the night and the high-pitched screaming had stopped.

Understanding Symptoms

Help your child identify the symptoms they are experiencing. The awareness they gain can help link physical reactions to a specific incident or memory about their traumatic experience. Physical reactions can become less frightening and dehabilitating if children understand their cause or meaning. Here's what you might say and do:

- Like hearts, it's normal for bodies to hurt sometimes, too. Even if you were not hurt physically, or even if your body has healed from injury, you may hold on to physical symptoms for a while.

- Sometimes our bodies hold on to memories just like our mind does.

- Symptoms will lessen over time.

- Where in your body does it hurt?

- Where in your body did you feel what happened?

- How did your body feel before, during, and after the event (Did you feel shaky, sick, numb, cold, hot, dizzy, dry mouth, etc.)?

- If your headache or stomachache (etc.) could talk, what would it say?
- What might help it feel better?
- What can I do to help?
- What makes it feel worse?
- It might help to write a letter to the stomachache (or other symptom) and talk to it for a while.
- Draw a picture of the dizziness (or other symptom).

Minimizing Stress

It's not realistic to think you will be able to alleviate all your child's stress after being impacted by trauma, but you can minimize it. Here's what to do:

- Increase rest and relaxation. Plan more time to read soothing books together; have your child soak in a warm bath with a new toy, soap, or special towel and washcloth set (perhaps with a favorite cartoon character on it); listen to soft music at naps and bedtime.

- Use nurturing touch. With all the warnings we must teach children around the kinds of unwanted and unsafe "touch" that are abusive, we can also help them understand the benefits of safe and nurturing touch. Nurturing touch can soothe, relax, and relieve stress. Similar to massage, but with a lighter touch, some children find comfort from having their backs, heads, or feet lightly stroked or "tickled."

- Keep routines as stable as possible.

- Keep daily schedules as nonhurried and nonrushed as possible.

- Maintain well-balanced meals and keep healthy snacks available.

- Stay in regular contact with your child's doctor. It's important that they stay in good health.

- Monitor television, radio, and movies for upsetting themes and stories.

- Offer increased comfort, physical support, and security. Sometimes hugging, touching, or holding is more than an older child wants or needs from you. Being present physically may be enough. Ask your child what they'd prefer.

- Play a new or familiar game.

It is important to be sensitive to children's physical complaints. Make note of any patterns that may be important for doctors, school nurses, or therapists to be aware of.

Professional Debriefing

Professional debriefing is first aid for the heart, mind, body, and soul. It is an immediate intervention that may help prevent the long-term complications that can result from unresolved trauma.

Debriefing an experience can help children begin to make sense of what happened. It is an opportunity for children to recall the various feelings, thoughts, and physical sensations experienced throughout the trauma. This process can bring into awareness the reactions that may have caused various symptoms. If Stacy had identified the details of her reactions early on, it is possible she could have been spared the dramatic physical symptoms she suffered.

When trauma impacts a number of people, as it did in Stacy's experience, a "critical incident debriefing group" is an important service professionals can offer to survivors, witnesses, and sometimes whole communities. Unlike general support groups, these are professionally led, one-time interventions usually conducted in small group settings. Professionals help traumatized people discuss, understand, and cope with what they've been through in a positive and supportive environment. Participants learn about the normal reactions to trauma and are given skills for coping with them. Together, the trauma survivors are given the opportunity to voluntarily talk about their experience within an educational and structured format.

Stacy's experience could have been different if she had participated in a debriefing group. It might have been valuable also for Stacy's friends, other customers, restaurant personnel, and even the witnesses in the parking lot. Other people in the community who had connections to the families and victims may have benefited, too.

Participating in a debriefing group as soon after a trauma as possible may help alleviate symptoms; however, it may too soon for some children to be able to talk about or hear from others what they experienced. A professional therapist can help you determine whether or not such a group would be beneficial to your child. If your child is offered this service, make sure the group is being facilitated by a qualified professional who has experience and training in leading debriefing groups.

Receiving skillful support immediately following trauma often prevents the need for extended therapy in the future.

When Art and Play Is Hard Work

For some children, play completely ceases following a trauma. Like Stacy, the energy and vitality they once had for games and make-believe play diminishes. Others reenact what happened through their play. According to child researcher Lenore C. Terr, post-traumatic play is a frequent and common manifestation of traumatic anxiety in children. She found that the sense of enjoyment that accompanies play is absent in post-traumatic reenactments (Terr 1981a). Play stops being fun. When this happens you may observe a sense of ongoing urgency and distress as traumatized children participate in art and play. Their actions may be repetitious and tense. Children may repeat and reenact the same ideas, feelings, or actions over and over again. Play and creative art no longer provide them with a source of relaxation and enjoyment.

If children are able to categorize people as good or bad, right or wrong, mean or nice, it simplifies life and increases their ability to feel prepared in the face of danger. Some children choose to align with the "bad guys" or the offenders responsible for the crime or trauma in their make-believe play. By "becoming" the person they fear the most, children can look for answers and try to figure out what makes people do bad things.

🐚 *As our work together continued, Stacy repeatedly drew pictures of the crime scene she witnessed. Over and over again in our sessions, she attempted to draw what she feared the most. She wanted to be able to pass the restaurant without feeling ill. By looking at the restaurant on paper, Stacy felt it might help prepare her for the real thing. Sometimes she felt dizzy seeing the restaurant and sometimes she didn't, but Stacy told me she wanted "to get it out" so she could see the restaurant without worrying about getting dizzy. As she drew, Stacy became visibly shaken. She did not want her art displayed on my office walls, quite unlike children who draw for a different purpose. Instead, one day she carefully folded up her drawing of the restaurant, pushed it across the table to me, and whispered, "I want you to keep it for me." Stacy asked if it could be tucked away in my wallet. She asked me to leave it there until she wanted it back.*

I supported Stacy's choice to "give it away" for a while. I complimented her ability to know what she needed to do. I assured her that when it was time to look at the picture of the restaurant again she would be able to. I explained that she could learn to accept her physical symptoms, even if the dizziness made her faint. For now she wanted to let go of the picture and stop redrawing it. I told Stacy I could hold on to it for as long as she needed, reassuring her that the picture did not worry or upset me. I told her I thought it was a very important drawing and that I felt honored to hold it for her.

When children don't appear to be having the fun they once did, here's what you might consider saying:

- Anything you want to play is okay as long as it's safe for you and everyone around you.

- It's normal to feel differently and to play differently for a while. Friends might tell you how you've changed and that you aren't as much fun as you used to be, but in time they'll have fun with you again.

- You may think you aren't fun to be with either, and in time you'll rediscover how much fun you are.

- It's hard for most kids to have fun after they've seen/heard/ found out about something happening like you have.

- Play will feel fun again in time.

- Sometimes it's important to play and draw pictures with a counselor who understands how to help you cope with what you've been through.

You cannot always control what is imposed on your kids. But you can allow for the free expression of what they see in the world around them. And you can be their companions as they attempt to deal with their anxiety and make sense of senseless events. It's important to accept all facets of children's play, and when possible, help them come to an understanding of the connection between their play and the trauma.

Trained counselors know how to use play and art so that it can lead to change and help free a child of distress. Professional intervention is needed when play and art are persistently unsatisfying and anxiety producing. Without help, repetitive themes in play or drawings can escalate distress and increase symptoms of stress and anxiety.

Physical Reactions

Regression

Fear may take the form of nightmares or increased anxiety. Children may go back to earlier behaviors in an attempt to comfort themselves and feel more secure. Their behaviors and needs may become regressed. Children may start wetting their beds, sucking their thumbs, and refusing to dress and feed themselves the way they did prior to the trauma. This form of regression is a natural response to childhood stress and fear. Adolescents may regress to an earlier state of development also. Their behaviors often become more childlike and immature.

A traumatized five-year-old girl I worked with found her pacifier and began using it again. For three weeks, a seven-year-old client crawled into bed with his parents in the middle of the night. In both cases, these children were not punished and they were not made to feel ashamed for their behaviors. Providing increased security is crucial at this time. Lovingly and patiently, these children were guided back to their former ways of being. As security increased, both children relaxed and returned to their former routines. Life was possible again without a pacifier and nights alone in bed were again the norm.

A change to earlier, more immature behaviors can become annoying and hard on everyone in the family. Rather than get angry or make children feel ashamed, gently explain to family members that a traumatized child's behaviors are different from what they usually are and sometimes it's hard to know how to respond, but that it's important to be understanding.

Children will give up what they don't need when they're ready. Parents need to help teach their children how to be ready. You can do that by helping them accept all of their behaviors and by letting them hear your confidence in their ability to change. You may say something like, "I can see how nice it feels to have your pacifier back right now. I know one day you'll decide you don't need it again, like you did before. When you feel older again, it won't even matter not to have it! Let me know when I should put it back in a special place where we can save it for you."

Dependency

Children who have high dependency needs are terrified of living life alone. After a trauma, it may feel intolerable, if not impossible, for kids to function independently from you, even when they had been prior to the trauma. Children may feel unable to fall asleep without your presence, make decisions without your input, or complete any simple task without your assistance.

Disturbing news and awareness of new information surrounding a trauma may also ignite dependency needs, requiring increased physical comfort and support. This is especially common when legal proceedings are taking place and the family is in upheaval. Sometimes offenders are not kept behind bars. This information is understandably upsetting to everyone and will intensify your child's fears for safety. Be prepared for times when your child feels extra clingy.

In a developmental age where a child's need for greater separation from family is increasing, it may be especially difficult for your child to suddenly become very dependent on you. A sudden need to know your constant whereabouts and plans for the day may cause feelings of embarrassment in an older child. These conflicting needs sometimes create confusion for kids and parents alike.

Stacy expressed embarrassment and shame around needing to be close to her parents all the time. She knew her behavior was different, but her fear of fainting without her parents there to assist her was more frightening than the discomfort of appearing "babyish." Her symptom of fainting caused her to feel out of control and helpless in the same way she was during the shooting. More than anything else, she wanted her parents nearby by for her sense of safety and security.

When I returned home from the hospital following a car crash I was injured in, I stayed awake as long as I could possibly manage. Just as I would begin the slow ascent into sleep, it would happen again: blinding headlights, the sound and feel of crushing metal against my chest. It no longer mattered that I was a teenager trying to separate and become more independent. To be able to sleep I needed a hand to hold to stay grounded. I needed my mom.

Dependency needs are not permanent. Once children find their bearings they will continue on the road to their developing independence. Dependency reactions are another natural and temporary outcome of trauma.

Separation

Two of the greatest fears children have following trauma are separation and abandonment. Separation anxiety is likely to be greatly heightened when an unexpected situation occurs that may threaten the safety and unity of the family (Bowlby 1973). Now more than ever, your children are depending on you to be there for them. They may worry every time you are not physically present. One child who was fearful of another burglary striking his household yelled for his mom whenever she left the room he was in. His constant need to hear her voice and know her exact location prevented him from dissolving into tears and becoming overwhelmed with panic. He did not want to be alone and unprotected "when the bad guys came back."

At home, your child's need to be continually reassured of your presence may become tiring. It may be difficult to leave the room for even a moment. You may wonder if this is okay or acceptable. It is absolutely normal. Most kids are simply letting you know in the only way they can that they have increased needs for safety, care, and nurturing. Once security has been reestablished you will see children bounce back again. This takes time and patience. Children will go at their own pace.

Separation anxiety will be evident in children who are fearful for their safety and for yours. It will take time for bonds to be reestablished and security to be trusted. Responding to their anxiety is very important. If you meet children's needs early on they will adjust better over time.

How to Help

Here are some suggestions on how to help your child cope with the discomfort of separating from you:

- Initially, remain in the company of your children as much as possible.

- Never sneak away from children or try to distract them from noticing the disappearance of someone else.

- When you must leave children before they are ready, be honest about it. Prepare them ahead of time; tell them your specific plan for who will care for them and what they will do. Talk about when you will return.

- Many children find it comforting when a parent or loved one leaves an important belonging with them until they return. This might be a wallet, scarf, coin purse, picture, jewelry, or other familiar object they know well.

- Telephone calls can also bring needed reassurance while you are away.

The key to resolving separation anxiety is to give children permission to have it. Let your child be your guide.

Sleep Disturbances

Nighttime is a vulnerable time for children. Fears and complaints often escalate. Separating from the family to go to bed is especially uncomfortable and frightening for traumatized children.

Establishing nighttime rituals can help. Plan special activities for your child before bedtime:

- Select special books to read that are only brought out at bedtime.

- Listen to music and story tapes that are selected as bedtime treats. (Harp music and sounds of the ocean and nature are popular choices.)

- Use night-lights if they are helpful.

- Prepare a warm bath for your child.

- Use relaxation exercises (e.g., have children focus on their breathing and imagine heaviness in their limbs and over their eyes).

- Use nurturing touch.

- Let your child sleep with a pet if that is comforting to them.

- Encourage children to compose letters, poetry, and/or a diary or journal.

- Make a planning list together for something your child is looking forward to (e.g., a birthday party, vacation, holiday, or gift list).

- If bedtime can be special time with you or other loved ones, it will help alleviate related anxiety.

Nightmares

Most parents are familiar with the heart-stopping experience of hearing their child scream out in the night. Terrifying dreams can leave children shaken, tearful, and afraid to go back to sleep. Nightmares may run like a movie, replaying the trauma that's on their mind or contain frightening images like monsters, witches, or dragons. If children can recall what they were dreaming about, let them tell you about it. Look for ways to help them overcome their fears.

For example, some children are particularly helped by "magic tools." One boy I know kept "dragon spray" by his bed. Before he went to sleep each night he used a bottle filled with water to spray a protective mist of dragon poison around himself. He stopped using it when he knew he had successfully warded off all the dragons that were once "after him."

Expression diffuses fear. Sharing frightening feelings around dreams can help kids reestablish what's real and what's not. They can be reminded of what could never really happen and why. If they dreamt of the trauma they experienced, they can be reminded that what happened is over. It helps to talk a dream through and see it for the fantasy it is.

Even though bad dreams and nightmares are frightening, you can tell children what's good about having them. Help kids understand that all dreams, even scary ones, can help them let go of what scares them the most. Explain that dreams can show the secret worries and troubling fears they may be holding but don't know what to do with. Tell them that dreams can help show them what they might need to talk more about.

You can also let children know that sometimes they can change what they dream about. Help your child take control of scary dreams, especially recurring ones, by encouraging them to create a new ending or change it in any way they would like to. Here are some ways they can do this:

- They can tell you about a new and improved ending or scenario.

- They can show you by acting out a new and different ending.

- They can draw a picture.

- They can re-write the dream and change the ending.

Help your child complete these activities in as much detail as they can by asking questions about everything they tell you. Let them add humor and silly, impossible outcomes if they want to. This exercise can help children create a sense of their own power and control over scary thoughts and memories. It often changes the dream as well. If children can regain a sense of confidence in one more area they feel vulnerable and helpless in, it will help them move further along the path to healing.

Returning to the Scene of Trauma

Returning to the scene of a crime or trauma is one of the most difficult and excruciating experiences a child will endure. Witnesses to trauma can experience the same reactions to the event that a direct victim does when they are reminded of what they experienced.

The first time I returned to the curve in the road where a drunk driver hit me in a head-on crash, I was not prepared for what happened to me that day anymore than I was the night of the crash. My hands grew wet, my body began shaking, my breathing became shallow, and I was certain from the images that flashed in my mind that every car that passed was headed straight for my windshield again.

For many children, returning to the scene of a crime or trauma means going back to their own home or school. Many develop chronic stomachaches, headaches, and vague physical complaints before and after they return to the site where they were traumatized.

Assuming it is now safe, should you insist that your child quickly return to the scene? Will it help them more or less in the long run? How do you know what is truly in your child's best interest or what may lead to further distress?

The Decision to Go Back

Every situation is different, and so is the child who experienced it. You will want to listen and be sensitive to hearing what your child's needs are. They may be very different from what other children are doing, and they deserve to feel okay about that. Children are empowered by your respect for their needs.

After a trauma, reestablishing regular routines as quickly as possible can be beneficial for kids. Sometimes, however, adults can expect too much, too soon from children. Change takes time, and children need time to adjust to their experience. Most people need some distance from trauma before they can feel ready to be close to it again. In the meantime, much work can be done to help your child prepare for a return to normalcy.

Recommendations

Before you and your children make the decision to return to the scene, consider these recommendations:

- Reestablish regular routines within your home and family first.

- Offer comfort, safety, and nurturing every chance you get.

- Reassure your child that their reactions are completely normal to have after a trauma.

- Remind them that their distress will lessen over time.

- Regardless of where the trauma occurred, ask children how they might know when they are ready to return to daily routines at home or school. How do they imagine they might think and feel when they're ready to return to the scene?

Preparation

Prepare your child for returning to the scene. Here's what you can do:

- Talk openly about how it might feel, what they might think about, what they will do, where they will go, and how they will cope.

- Help your children identify what they heard, saw, and were doing in the minutes before the trauma. Then explain that they can prepare themselves before doing/seeing/hearing similar things that may trigger strong reactions.

- In detail, talk about what things might remind them of what happened and when they can expect to see or hear those reminders. For example, if the trauma happened at school, there might be reminders like bells ringing, doors opening or shutting, cars backfiring, children yelling or laughing, clocks ticking, pencils being sharpened, etc.

- Have a plan if symptoms of stress become too difficult for children to bear. What can they do, where can they go, and who can they tell? Make sure they will have a way to cope with whatever comes up.

When the Trauma Scene Is School

If the trauma occurred at your child's school, the first few days back will be especially difficult. Acknowledge this openly. There is no way you can make it different. Help your child accept the fact that it will be difficult for *everyone*.

How School Staff Can Help

Staff at schools that have suffered tragedies can help facilitate the healing process in many ways. Here are some suggestions for your child's school, which you may want to request/suggest:

- If possible, schools should make available professionally led debriefing groups to *everyone* impacted by the trauma. These should take place as soon as possible following a tragedy and before school reopens. All school personnel need to be invited (i.e., janitors, cafeteria workers, office personnel, and administrative staff). Sometimes the principal and other administrators are so busy supporting and leading the staff that they don't have time to take care of themselves. Find ways to help support all the leaders in the crisis. For example, provide nourishing snacks, offer to run errands, step in whenever you can to give them a break, and/or ask what you can do to help. Most importantly, acknowledge their role and find ways to show your appreciation.

- Schools can immediately distribute flyers with referrals for counseling support.

- It can be helpful to open the school for a few hours before the reopening day and allow children to return with you and other family members for support. Volunteers may want to hand out ribbons, flowers, or other meaningful items that symbolize the loss and the hope there is for healing.

- To counteract the shock and numbness children are feeling, special activities can be created for everyone to participate in. Children might express feelings through posters and paintings. Participate with them if they'd like you to.

- Suggest that your school allow everyone to freely express their thoughts and feelings on a "memory wall" or line a fence with memories and special tributes. Create a place for all to pay their respects and spend time remembering.

- Start a "teddy bear campaign." Encourage the public to donate new teddy bears or stuffed animals for the children. The media can publicize your request and help show children how many people care. Let the community give and reach out in ways that will help you comfort your children and all those suffering.

- In time, adults can assist schools in creating opportunities for renewing innocence through events that balance pain with the joy still found in life. A school-wide talent show or carnival or a community-wide picnic can provide opportunities for everyone to come together in a different way.

- Special memorials can be planned as a tribute to the victims and in remembrance of what everyone has suffered. Some schools plan nondenominational services to acknowledge the spiritual impact of the event.

- Schools have the unique ability to bring everyone together at once. They can provide opportunities to explain the wide range of normal reactions you and your children can expect to experience. All of you can feel reassured when school personnel explain the measures being taken to prevent such a trauma from happening again.

You might suggest to your school staff that the first two days back to school be designated as special days for healing and nurturing. Expectations for anything more will not be helpful for most. Through the weeks ahead, parents and teachers will need to expect a range of responses from the children affected.

When Friends Are Reminders of Trauma

Friends and classmates may represent a type of reminder to each other of what happened. Whoever children were with when the trauma happened will likely trigger memories somewhere inside them. Most children don't understand their feelings of wanting to avoid certain friends and will fear being together for this reason. Others will feel superstitious about being with the same people, in the same place, or doing the same things, for fear the trauma will happen again.

When my friend lay unconscious and near death in an intensive care unit hospital bed, I blacked out every time the phone rang. I was injured and heavily medicated but able to recuperate at home from the car crash we were in together. I feared the phone call that would tell me she had died, but she recovered and was sent home several weeks later. We talked very little over the phone and made no attempts to see each other.

We were fortunate that one of our parents sensed something was wrong. My friend's mom wasn't sure why, but she knew we needed to be together and arranged for us to meet. We were tense. Secretly, we both dreaded the meeting. We didn't have any logical explanation for why we didn't want to see each other, we just knew we didn't. I was embarrassed and ashamed of myself for feeling the way I did.

After fifteen seconds of awkwardness we both suddenly knew. We looked at each other and confessed that we were afraid of each other. We had thoughts of something else bad happening to us if we were together again. And then we laughed until we cried. How silly, we decided, to think our friendship was somehow "jinxed."

We spent many hours trying to decide if there was a purpose for our experience and why it happened. We examined our faith and talked about the spiritual experiences we both felt that night. But there was something else neither of us could articulate yet. We were trying to avoid the "traumatic reminder" we were for each other. We were afraid seeing one another would trigger more intrusive thoughts, feelings, memories, and bad dreams. We didn't want to remember what we had been through during the worst moments of our experience. We didn't realize that trying to avoid reminders wouldn't help. I learned through this encounter that it is only when you *let* yourself be reminded that you are able to diffuse the impact of these experiences.

If you sense or notice that your children are avoiding certain people or places, talk to them about it. Encourage children to spend time with friends who shared their experience, even if at first it's difficult to be with them again. What you might say to help:

- Just because you went through a trauma together does not mean your friendship is "jinxed" or "bad luck."

- It's natural to feel nervous about being together. It's normal to want to avoid being with people or going to places that remind you of what happened.

- You might be afraid that seeing your friend will cause you to have more intrusive thoughts, feelings, memories, or bad dreams, but trying to avoid the situation won't help. I will be there to help you through it, if you decide you need me.

- When you *let* yourself be reminded, you may find that the experience won't continue to feel as frightening.

- You might find that you will be relieved to be together again. It's difficult to stop being friends with people you care about and who care about you. Dealing with your difficult feelings about being together is easier than losing a friend.

- Once you've had the chance to spend time together, your friendship will mean more than just the traumatic experience you shared.

Anniversary Dates: Prepare to Remember

When you experience trauma, you are never the same again. Over the past twenty-five years, my friend and I have noticed every March 22 that passes—the anniversary of the car crash that we were in together. We have stopped each year on that date to reflect on how thankful we are to be alive. We've remained close despite the miles between us and infrequent contact. That night we became bonded in a way that only people who have survived and recovered through a trauma together can. It remains a bittersweet chapter in our lives, one we were both able to learn and grow from.

Ask any survivor when they were traumatized and you will likely hear an exact date and time. Anniversary dates are powerful reminders and evoke many different reactions in people. Seasonal reminders and the time of year can trigger profound physical sensations. Adults and children alike take in all the details around them. During times of traumatic stress, all the senses are heightened so that sights, sounds, and smells that wouldn't normally be noticed are remembered. Many details aren't identified until long after the event, when they seem to come out of nowhere. Preparing children for anniversary dates can help them take control of their reactions.

A student asked me once, "Why do they call it an anniversary anyway? An anniversary means something happy, not sad." I told her it can also mean something important to remember. However you choose to think about it, an anniversary date of a trauma can be an important time to reflect, honor, and respect the event that changed your child's life. Many people use the day to help them move further along in their search for acceptance of what happened. Some families and schools attach new and different meanings to the anniversary date. One family planned a special trip for the anniversary of their trauma. They went to a tropical island they had never been to and relaxed and played. They created a new memory to replace the old. Their anniversary date no longer represented just the trauma.

Anniversaries can become a celebration of survival or simply another year further away from what happened. Perhaps it will mean another year closer to regaining normalcy and healing. Others need to remember that date for exactly what it was: a tragedy and loss they will never forget, a day when disaster or an act of human cruelty took the lives of people they loved and will always remember.

Give children time, prepare them for the tough stuff ahead, and be there to help them face their "dragons."

☞ *I was certain that before Stacy could return to a normal life she would need to understand why she was fainting. To do that she would need to remember more of what happened. I believed, as I always do after a trauma, that a person's symptoms always make sense in view of what happened. I believed Stacy's fainting spells were happening for a good reason.*

I referred Stacy to a trusted colleague who was a certified hypnotherapist. I explained to Stacy that I believed good counselors needed to be good detectives sometimes. I explained that he might be able to help us uncover some important clues. Fortunately she enjoyed Nancy Drew mysteries as much as I had, so we set out to solve what she titled "The Mystery of the Dizzy Debutante," and she agreed it had the makings of a great story if we could give it a real ending.

With Stacy and her parent's permission, the hypnotherapist was able to help her remember details of the experience which until that point she had been unable to recall. Through hypnosis we learned that during the shooting, Stacy had visually focused all her attention on a pizza delivery truck in the parking lot across from the restaurant. By doing this she had effectively tuned the rest of the world out. She did not hear the screaming, crying, broken glass, or sirens. From then on, she became faint every time she saw one of the popular trucks. Seeing them physically took her back to the shock and terror her body experienced. The trucks were commonly seen around town, on television, in the newspaper, even on ads in an elevator. No place was safe from being reminded.

Stacy retained a physical memory even when she consciously had "forgotten" most of what she saw, heard, and felt. Fainting was a symptom directly related to the trauma. In her attempt to block out everything happening around her, Stacy focused on the furthest thing she could see from her terror. She was able to eventually understand that focusing all of her attention on the truck helped her believe that the horror wasn't really happening. She wanted to be where the truck was parked instead of where she was.

Stacy told me she didn't want to know when it would happen—the moment she would be shot. People were screaming, and she knew she couldn't get away. Once we discovered the meaning it held, she was able to accept the full range of her experience. Remembering helped her make sense of her body's normal reactions. Fainting was no longer frightening. She felt compassion for the symptom. She knew it was her body's way of coping with something unbearable. She understood at last that she wasn't "crazy."

It took time for Stacy to face her fears of seeing the pizza trucks. First, she practiced seeing one in her mind without feeling light-headed. We looked at pictures of the trucks and ads in the paper, and she was able to remain relaxed. In time, Stacy asked for her picture of the restaurant that was still tucked away in my wallet. She opened it and learned how to look at it and remain calm.

   Step-by-step, Stacy learned to no longer associate these terrifying minutes with seeing the pizza truck or the restaurant where it all happened. It would always be remembered, but the memory no longer had the power to incapacitate her. More importantly, the memory lost the power to cause a frightening physical symptom she thought she had no control over. Before too long, Stacy returned to her normal activities and grew increasingly confident being apart from her parents again.

   In one of our last appointments together, we ordered pizza to celebrate her recovery and survivorship. Of course it could only be the pizza delivered by the truck we worked so hard to find! When it arrived at my office, Stacy did not faint or become dizzy. Her only physical symptom that afternoon was the result of eating too much pizza.   ❧

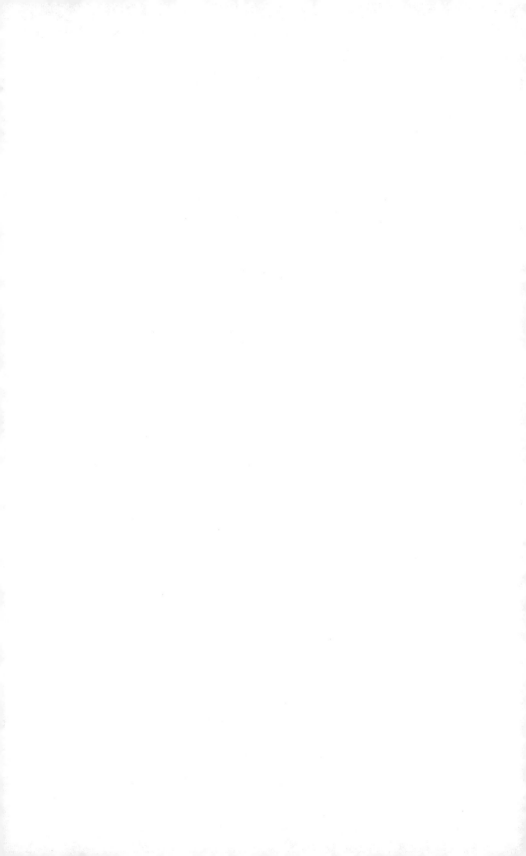

4

Healing the Soul

"If there's a God, why did this happen?"

The last time Kevin was with his grandmother, he complained that she was "on his case." Like most twelve-year-olds, he was tired of being told what to do and tired of being treated "like a baby." That afternoon, his grandmother was critical of what he had eaten, what time he had gotten to bed the night before, and the way he was dressed. Most of the time she was okay though, even fun, and Kevin knew she meant well. He usually managed to be polite even when he didn't feel like it. He only wished he had been polite that day. Instead, Kevin lost his temper and yelled things he later wished he hadn't.

That evening, Kevin was on his bike when he saw police cars and an ambulance parked on his grandparents' street. Out of curiosity he rode to see what all the excitement was about. He was confused when he saw long strips of yellow tape surrounding his grandparents' home and stunned to see police officers walking back and forth through their front door. A neighbor boy told Kevin that there was a dead body in the bag they carried out on a stretcher. Kevin had no memory of his frantic ride home.

Kevin's grandmother was shot in the head at close range while sitting in bed reading. His grandfather was convicted of the crime.

Kevin came to my office because his parents insisted he talk to someone. They were worried about him because he had grown increasingly quiet and withdrawn since the murder. In my office, Kevin was polite and patient, but he didn't want to be in counseling. He wanted to talk about his feelings of guilt even less.

Kevin said counseling wasn't anything he really needed. So we played checkers instead. We played so many rounds that I began seeing black and red circles and squares after our sessions. One week when I told him this he laughed and we played a game of Yahtzee for a change. It was this change that helped Kevin begin to express his thoughts and feelings.

Kevin liked games and his grandmother did, too. He told me he stayed up until three in the morning playing Yahtzee with his grandmother one weekend when his parents were out of town. He said she made games fun. She knew how to "kid around" and make him laugh. He continued sharing his fondest memories of her. He told me about the special trips they took to all-you-can-eat buffets, the chocolate chip cookies she'd make at his request, the nickname "graham cracker" he had given her when he was three. He talked about their trips to water-slide parks and to their favorite restaurant for barbecued ribs. He said some of his best memories were of times with his grandma and grandpa. And then Kevin asked me, "If there's a God, why did this happen?"

I told Kevin that I thought his question was an important one to ask. I let him know I understood why he would feel so confused about the existence of God. I agreed that there were many things that were hard for us to understand, and I explained that often there are no easy answers to some of the questions we face. We discussed many possibilities, but ultimately, through the process of his healing, Kevin would need to answer his own question.

Kevin's upbringing included church. His faith had taught him to love and respect his family. It had taught him to celebrate life after death. It taught him the importance of forgiveness. Kevin believed he had failed at everything he was supposed to have learned. He questioned all he knew and said he didn't know what he believed anymore. Kevin felt betrayed by God, betrayed by his grandfather, and betrayed by himself. He felt he deserved to be punished for the cruel things he had said to his grandmother. He suffered deep remorse for not having the chance to take it all back.

Kevin was full of rage, shock, and confusion. For the first time in his life he hated his grandfather. Kevin had never loved and hated someone so much at the same time as he did his grandfather. He struggled with questions about why and how his grandfather could have taken the life of the person he had been married to for nearly fifty years. He thought his grandfather had loved her deeply. He thought they were so happy. Kevin felt he no longer stood on the firm foundation he was raised on. It had slipped out from under him in an emotional earthquake.

Kevin had a wound so deep, he thought he had lost his soul. In the months ahead, I learned what a powerful medicine faith could be. It would help Kevin discover that not only was the foundation under him still intact, it could also grow stronger. &

Trauma Hurts the Soul

Trauma attacks the spirit. It can kill hopes, dreams, and a sense of meaning in life. It's common for children to experience a spiritual crisis as a result of a traumatic experience.

Issues of life and death and facing one's mortality are bound to raise painful questions, doubts, and fears. If children are supported in their search to find spiritual comfort and understanding, these fears can be resolved and may even lead to new spiritual growth and development.

Not all counseling or therapy work includes a spiritual component, but I believe there is rich opportunity and healing to be gained for both adults and children from exploring the depths of the soul in the midst of suffering.

The soul needs healing too.

The Search for Meaning

Having a sense of purpose and meaning in life can help you transcend painful or confusing experiences. Spiritual exploration is a natural and necessary step in looking for meaning in tragedy and restoring hope and trust in the future. It's an important part of resolving a life-altering experience.

For many adults, the search is twofold: there is the desire to understand the meaning of life and also to live a life of meaning. In their own way children search, too. They may wonder about personal and cultural beliefs, God, or a philosophy about life in relation to the tragedy they faced. They may wonder why bad things happen in the world and why "bad people" sometimes make them happen.

Your own beliefs, philosophy, or religion may be well defined and structured or loosely formed and constantly evolving, but the search for truth and meaning seems to be universal, even for children.

Suffering

It's hard to make sense out of suffering. Holocaust survivor Viktor E. Frankl's book *Man's Search for Meaning* (Frankl 1963) suggests that it is through suffering that we can reach a greater spiritual depth and find meaning in life. It has been said that "there are no atheists in a foxhole." The threat of death and the experience of trauma quickly challenges belief systems and causes most people to reevaluate their ideas about the meaning of life. It is an experience that can be personally compelling and life changing. For some, it is the unwanted and unwarranted suffering they endured that enables them to connect with something deeper inside themselves.

Trauma can change children in subtle ways or profoundly alter the direction of their lives. Some people say they appreciate life more and that life is richer because of what they learned through their experiences.

Of course, trauma isn't the only way to grow appreciative of life, but if it is an experience you and your family had to endure, you can choose to find a way to reconcile what you went through and so can your child. You don't always find answers in your quest for spiritual resolution, but sometimes it's enough to find relief.

Spiritual Beliefs

Your spiritual beliefs provide a framework for the way you live and for the choices you make. Your belief system may even help you explain tragedies in life when they happen to you or others. Children talk about spiritual beliefs for the same reason. They are often looking for a new framework to build around their experience, one that will help them make sense of what seemed so senseless.

A traumatic experience often calls spiritual beliefs into question. When this happens beliefs may be strengthened or shattered. They may be a source of comfort or despair. Regardless, you can help your children find inner peace as you guide them through the spiritual obstacle course they may be facing.

The road to inner peace is a different journey for each child, but suffering must be relieved before any child is able to get there.

Trauma can exercise beliefs by forcing you to use and rely on them, but even if yours have been strengthened, helping your child find relief from what happened is not always easy.

I have worked with families from a variety of spiritual backgrounds, but I cannot tell you how to respond to every question of faith or beliefs. I can tell you the children who were given a foundation of beliefs they could embrace and depend on, moved through their suffering easier. The families of these children had four things in common:

- They recognized their need for a spiritual life.
- They modeled their personal beliefs for each other.
- Spiritual discipline was taught based on love, not fear.
- They practiced their beliefs within a supportive structure or organization.

James Garbarino, author of *Raising Children in a Socially Toxic Environment,* asserts that strong families are anchored in a sense of purpose—usually religious or spiritual in its foundation. A leading authority on at-risk children and youth, Garbarino believes there needs to be open acknowledgment of the spiritual side of life and its protective power in the lives of youth (Garbarino 1995). Andrew Weaver found studies to document the fact that spirituality (in the form of nonpunitive religion) exerts an anchoring effect on kids including a better response to trauma. Traumatized teens involved in religious institutions feel more social support, are more likely to find meaning in the event, and experience lower distress and faster recovery than other teens (Weaver 1998, Garbarino 1999).

Children who hold beliefs that are meaningful to them have one more resource available to them in their healing process. Those I have worked with who have used their spiritual beliefs to help them heal often say it was the reason they got better.

Most adults will draw from their own upbringing to respond to their children's spiritual needs. The way your family approached learning about spiritual beliefs help shape who you are now and what you believe. Like your parents, you will have an influence on the spiritual and moral development of your child. Positive or negative, your attitudes and outlook on life will affect your child's.

The foundation of beliefs and standards you establish may help support your children as they struggle to understand a traumatic event. It can give children a place to stand while they look for balance and security.

In times of trauma, a foundation to stand on can be like an island in the middle of a turbulent sea. When you are grounded in a philosophy or approach that reflects your values you can successfully guide, teach, direct, and protect your children. Values are at the core of your foundation of beliefs.

How do you confidently share the foundation of your beliefs to help your child through times of traumatic injury? How do you do this if you didn't have a spiritual foundation before the trauma? And what if you want to help your child build a spiritual foundation apart from an organized or structured organization? Whether you have a foundation, are seeking a foundation, or prefer a secular belief system or ideology, sharing a foundation of values with your children can strengthen your family. One way you might begin is to help children recognize and understand that values and beliefs are expressed through the behaviors people choose. You might begin doing this by identifying the behaviors and actions demonstrated by those who responded to the trauma and assisted those in need. Explain the impact their behaviors had on others and on the situation as a whole. Ask children to think about what other behaviors and actions they've seen since. Here are a few examples to help you get started:

- Point out the favors friends and family have done for you since the trauma. Talk about similar favors you have done for others when they needed help.

- Talk about acts of generosity that you have seen in the news, at your child's school, or in your community.

- Show appreciation for helpfulness. Talk about why a behavior was especially helpful or needed at any point during or after the traumatic event.

- Tell or read a bedtime story that illustrates an important value or standard. Discuss the consequences of the choices characters make in the story and how it affects those around them. Talk about any choices that were made in relation to the trauma and the consequences those choices had on others.

- Pay attention to kindness. Notice out loud when you see, hear, or experience it from anyone through out the healing process.

With a strong foundation to guide them, kids stand an excellent chance of rejecting violence, growing more resilient to future stress, and embracing those behaviors that heal rather than hurt. A strong spiritual foundation gives your child something solid to stand on for life.

Spiritual Confusion

Many of the ideas and beliefs children held before a tragic incident may seem confusing or untrue to them following it. They may feel spiritually alone and abandoned. They may see life as scary instead of safe, realizing that bad things can happen even when you're good and thinking that whoever or whatever is in control of the world is mean instead of nice. Perhaps your child came face-to-face with death. They may have learned for the first time that dying means you can never come back and that even people they love and need can die.

Some children are forced to face these cold hard facts before they are developmentally ready. Spiritual confusion is uncomfortable and often frightening. It is important to respect whatever your child's spiritual experience has been.

I was about ten when a woman approached me on the sidewalk in front of my home early one evening. She looked peculiar to me. When she motioned to me to come over to her I went up to her out of curiosity. Her crazed eyes were fixated on the roof of our house. I saw nothing there, so I stared back into her big green eyes trying to figure out what her problem was. It seemed to me she wasn't completely "with it," but she was intent to tell me something very important and I was determined to wait until she got it out. She finally asked if my father was home. She said she needed to tell him what she saw. She described to me what she wanted him to know. It was a "vision," she said. She saw an old man over our house with round wire-frame glasses with a smile and a "twinkle" in his eye. "He came to say good-bye," she said. She told me he wanted us to know he loved us and that he blessed our home before he left.

It was my Grandpa Snow. My father's stepdad, who we lovingly referred to as "Pop." The lady left as quickly as she came. I never saw her again. But soon after the phone rang. It was a long-distance call from Rochester, Minnesota, telling us Pop had died earlier that evening.

Aside from the fact that I thought the woman was peculiar, the whole experience seemed normal enough to me, but I could tell by the reactions of the grown-ups around me that it wasn't. I tried to understand what it all meant, but no one could explain it to me. Pop loved us, I thought. Of course he would come and tell us good-bye. I had no idea that most people did not have this kind of experience when people they loved died.

For many years after whenever I heard that someone I knew had died, I worried when they might make their "appearance." I didn't mind other people seeing "dead people," but I wasn't sure I was ready to see one myself. My spiritual confusion resulted in a fear of "ghosts" that no one realized. It also resulted in a sense of excitement for the idea of a life in the "hereafter." The adults around me didn't have a clue how that evening had impacted my spiritual development.

Well-meaning adults may intentionally or unintentionally ignore the spiritual concerns and questions that have been awakened in their children since a trauma. Even if you're confused about what to say, remaining silent suggests to your child that spiritual issues are not worth exploring and not important to their well-being. A child's recovery from trauma is likely to be inhibited and healing may be incomplete when any of the following happen:

- Adults tease and/or discount children's spiritual feelings, beliefs, fears, or questions.

- Adults lecture in a way that prevents children from finding their own truth and reaching their own conclusions.

- Parents attempt to change their children's views or thinking.

- Parents are too distracted to really hear what their children are saying.

- Parents assume their child is too young to understand or have a spiritual life.

If children get the message that spiritual questions are not okay to discuss, they may choose to ignore their thoughts and feelings and lose a significant opportunity for further healing. Help them understand that everyone has questions and fears, especially after a trauma. Share with them your own childhood questions and fears. The openness you communicate may help your child move freely through spiritual confusion rather than forget or suffer alone with it. Self-expression is a fundamental need of the soul.

Maria felt spiritually strengthened as a result of her experience, but spiritual confusion was a prominent concern for Lisset and Stacy. In their own ways, all three girls went down into the "foxhole" and came out changed.

After Maria witnessed the fatal stabbing of her baby-sitter (chapter 1), she told me she prayed whenever she felt scared. She said her baby-sitter would have told her that was the right thing to do. Maria told me that when she prayed it made her feel brave. Maria made it clear to everyone around her that her strength and ability to testify so successfully in court came from the faith she said she gained from this traumatic experience. Supporting Maria's beliefs helped her to successfully heal.

After Lisset's home was broken into by a frightening stranger (chapter 2), she questioned her beliefs. She told me, "I feel sad because I used to be sure what I believed and now I'm not." Lisset suffered a spiritual loss as well as the loss of trust and sense of security in the world. She had many questions that needed to be asked. Providing an accepting, supportive atmosphere allowed her to feel safe enough to ask those questions. In time, she was able to resolve for herself the conflicts she faced. This insightful young girl told me, "Deep down, I know there is more good in the world than bad. If I stop seeing what's good, I'm never going to be happy."

After Stacy survived the restaurant shooting (chapter 3), she told me she wished she knew for sure whether God was real or not because what happened to her didn't make sense. She confided in me that she didn't understand why, if God was real, she would be protected when others were injured and killed. She said, "A part of me believes and a part of me doesn't. I want to believe, but I don't know how to anymore, after what happened."

Stacy was searching desperately for answers and a way back to the beliefs she held before the trauma. She felt unable to ask her parents for help because as she said, "They don't understand why it keeps bothering me." Counseling helped her gain confidence in her ability to question and explore. Stacy learned she would be taken seriously no matter what she brought to our sessions.   ✑

Caring for Your Children's Souls

Caring for your children's souls is as important as caring for their physical and emotional well-being. After trauma, nurturing your children's spiritual lives can help restore their heart, mind, body, and soul. As a parent or guardian, you have the opportunity to inspire and guide your child's soul in ways that only a close loved one can.

The Soul Needs Attention

There are three ways to help your child's soul receive the attention it needs right now. They are to *listen carefully, respond genuinely,* and *restore hope continuously.*

Listen Carefully

The first step in tending to your child's soul is to gain an understanding of the impact the trauma had on your child's spirit. In order to gain their trust, to be "let in" on the difficult struggles and pain, you must first listen respectfully, acknowledge and let them know their experiences are valid, and honor the unique perspectives they bring.

Gain your children's trust by listening with respect and giving your undivided attention while they talk. Give children time to speak about spiritual concerns, ideas, questions, and doubts, as well as personal experiences about the trauma they suffered. Your child needs time with you that is focused and uninterrupted. Children will gain strength, reassurance, and confidence in expressing beliefs and spiritual perspectives when they see that what they say truly matters to you.

When listening to your children's concerns or thoughts about spirituality, it's important that you acknowledge their feelings and validate what they are saying. When you listen, repeat to your children what you think you heard them say. Do this to be sure you are understanding correctly what they are telling or asking you. Let them know that what they share is valid and understandable. If you don't understand why they think something in particular, ask for help in understanding until you do.

During such discussions, help identify and clarify questions and answers. Share your best hunches about what it is your child means or is experiencing. You might say something like, "This is only a hunch, but I wonder if what you are really asking/wanting/needing/feeling is . . ."

If your children are silent about spiritually related questions and fears you can encourage them to talk, but don't push or insist that they speak about this aspect of the trauma in their life. Your children may not be at a point where it matters, or they may not be able to verbalize their feelings clearly. Continue to use these listening skills as a matter of routine. If it is too frightening for them to talk about, good listening in general on your part will help them build their confidence in disclosing difficult-to-discuss information.

Good listening lays the groundwork for your children's self-disclosure. In an atmosphere of respect and concern, they will feel free to explore spiritual questions and fears. They will also be more likely to listen when you share your beliefs and offer your guidance.

Respond Genuinely

Share your spiritual beliefs with your children. Begin by saying something like, "I believe . . . (explain specific values and religious or cultural beliefs)" and tell them why. When asked challenging questions like "Why is there suffering in the world?" be straightforward and honest. Give your answers in ways that kids will be able to understand and relate to. For example, "Sometimes suffering is unavoidable. Life can hurt, just like it can be fun. Life is always changing, just like you are physically. What's inside you might change too, but usually there are parts of people's thoughts and feelings that never change even through times of suffering."

Make a point to reframe experiences in a way that will help your child see value in living through the hard parts of life. For example, "Sometimes suffering can help you understand life in a way you never could before. If you can see something differently than you did before then you've learned from your suffering, and that is important. You may be able to use what you've learned sometime in the future or every day for the rest of your life."

For children who are silent about spiritual issues, it is still important to respond to them on this level. Without expecting a child to talk, you can still openly acknowledge and share all of what you believe to be true. Let them hear your willingness to teach and guide them.

Restore Hope Continuously

Children need hope to heal. When nothing seems to be getting better it is easy to lose all hope. Despair prevents you and your child from seeing the world clearly. Like a darkened lens over the eyes, it can change spiritual perspectives on life. Wearing it too long, you may think this way of seeing life is normal and forget the true picture.

Hope can overshadow even the deepest despair. Your children are depending on you to have a view of the world that will help them recover and hold on to hope. Here's what you might *say* to help restore your child's hope:

- It's hard for everyone to make sense of why something so bad happened.

- It's natural to question the beliefs you had before.

- Everything you believed might feel different now.

- Having something bad happen to you or around you doesn't mean you're bad.

- Life is full of experiences that will make you happy and make you sad. Happy times will come again.

- We all have a choice. We can choose to live in a way that shows our love for one another, or we can choose hurtful ways of being in the world.

- People aren't perfect and the world isn't perfect either. Earthquakes, floods, hurricanes, and tornadoes are all part of life, too.

Here's what you might *do* to help restore your child's hope:

- Change your lens and view of the world if you need to. Seek professional help to accomplish this if you aren't able to do this on your own.

- Use your beliefs or faith to teach your child about regaining hope.

- Help your children identify what they still have, as well as what is right about their lives and the world. This can help them balance their loss with positive perspectives.

Healing Exercises for the Soul

There is a time for hurt and pain and a time to let go of suffering. There are many approaches to help heal your child and family when you are all open and ready to let go of your suffering. You must ultimately teach your child how to allow the hurt to be taken away.

Meaningful Activities

You might encourage one of the following activities for your child's spiritual self-expression:

- Use prayer, meditation, and spiritual reflection to help transform hurt into healing. Encourage children to focus on whatever they want or need (i.e., strength, compassion, understanding, sleep, acceptance, relief from bad dreams, hope, love, support, and healing). Tell them to express the deepest yearnings of their heart and to be open to receiving comfort and guidance.

- Write in a journal whatever they are thinking about and describe the spiritual feelings they experienced or list the spiritual questions they have.

- Draw pictures of their spiritual thoughts, concerns, or feelings. (This is especially helpful for younger children who cannot write yet.)

- Write a letter to or a dialogue with whoever they have spiritual questions for.

- Write a letter to a person, deity, the event itself, or a part of themselves they are struggling with, such as feelings of fear or guilt.

- Talk to the strong and weak parts inside themselves.

- Talk to the obstacles in the way of their spiritual healing.

- Each night, have your children talk about the best part of their day and worst part of their day with you. Encourage them to give thanks or share your gratitude for the best and ask for help with the worst.

- Make a family gratitude list. At the end of each day share one thing each one of you is grateful for and write it on the list. Post it where the whole family can watch it grow.

The Wonder of Nature

A love and appreciation for nature can help restore the soul and soothe the spirit. Help your child discover the many simple but meaningful ways to spend time in spiritual reflection, prayer, or relaxation that is not necessarily structured or planned. Take a long walk and pay attention to the miracles in nature. This can help relieve stress and provide a new perspective on life. Some favorite ways to do this are to look at budding flowers, spider webs, stars in the night sky, shapes in clouds, a sunrise or sunset, birds, and the pounding waves at the ocean shore.

A Note to Religious Families

Trauma throws religious beliefs into question for many people. Your children may have become more active in their faith for consolation and comfort or felt their faith blocked by their resentment and doubts.

For many children, the burden of trauma is compounded by the burden of feeling abandoned by their God. There may be times as a parent when you too feel like giving up on divine providence. Children watch closely to see how the adults around them are coping. They need your help to know how to cope with spiritual feelings of betrayal and abandonment.

If you are finding it difficult to help your child over the rocky spiritual path you find yourselves on, you are not alone. Many adults feel outraged that their innocent child was not protected from life's cruelty. A supportive faith community, clergy, pastoral leader, or counselor may be able to help you reconcile your doubts and pain with your beliefs.

Questions of Faith

Questions of faith are a part of working through loss. Most children will need to explore their religious beliefs and express their questions and doubts after trauma has touched their lives. They may ask, "Where was God when this happened?" or "How do we know if there's life after death?" or "Why weren't people protected?" Children may experience anger and rage at the world, at you, at their God, and at their own faith.

It is important to accept children's acceptance or rejection of their beliefs with kindness and understanding. The following are suggestions of what you might say to offer help and reassurance:

- I hate what happened, too.

- It's normal to have doubts. It's hard to have faith when bad things happen.

- Sometimes kids find out that their faith grows stronger after a traumatic experience.

- It's normal to have mixed up feelings about what you believe or used to believe.

- Sometimes faith can be renewed or strengthened by others who come into your life just at the right time (police, doctors, counselors, clergy, nurses, family, friends, teachers, and anyone else who helps you heal).

Your Religious Community

While your religious community may be a source of great comfort, sometimes the reactions or responses your child and family receive add more stress than support. Religious organizations and communities may not always know how to help after a traumatic event.

Sometimes well-meaning people offer words of comfort that serve to exclude your present feelings and experience. Healing from trauma requires both children and adults to move through many legitimate and powerful feelings that must not be ignored.

Seek the support of others in your faith who have been through a traumatic event. You may find they can be more accepting of what you and your child are going through because they have been through a similar experience.

Renewing Your Child's Faith

If your children have lost faith, you can find ways to help guide them back to the assurance they once knew. You may want the clergy or the spiritual counselors in your religious community to meet with you, your child, or even your entire family. You may want to use the support of classes or worship services to help inspire your child. Consider reading stories or passages from your religious text that address what to do in times of tragedy or loss of faith. Discuss with your child the ways you see people coping with their feelings in the stories. There is a richness in many religious rituals. These can be an additional source of healing and spiritual comfort for children and their families.

It's okay not to know all the answers. Deal with the religious components to your faith as honestly as you can, and in your own time. Everyone's faith journey is different. Trauma may create new religious questions that will take time and patience for you to resolve.

Spiritual Dilemmas: Guilt, Anger, Forgiveness

Guilt

Guilt is an issue that comes up frequently for kids and often complicates their thoughts and feelings. Families will notice how feelings of guilt can block their child's healing process. It's easy to get stuck if the feelings aren't addressed. It is important to help your child resolve and look realistically at their feelings of guilt so they will be able to move past it.

Children may feel responsible for the trauma that disrupted their own life and their family's. They may worry that they said, thought, or wished something that caused it to happen. Some children believe the trauma was a way of being punished for being "bad" or unkind. Other children feel responsible for the family stress and chaos the trauma created.

Do your children feel responsible for what happened in any way? It's important to find out and respond accordingly. Here's how to begin:

- Ask them if they feel like they did anything wrong to cause the trauma.

- Listen carefully to the reasons your child feels responsible. Be careful not to try to talk children out of their feelings. Let them tell you about their feelings and respond only when they are finished talking. Make sure you are clear about their reasons and understand their feelings before you try to help them see another perspective.

- Explain and clarify all the facts of what happened (or at least as much as you know).

- Help your child understand that no one could have prevented what happened. You can help them see why they couldn't have stopped the trauma. For example, you could say, "You don't have special powers to see into the future. No one knew what was going to happen," or "Children are not able to stop the force of an adult," or "It was impossible for any one person to stop what happened."

- If your child continues to feel responsible you might say, "The crime or trauma was not your fault. I understand you feel the way you do, but the truth is you are not to blame. It's very important that you not blame yourself or anyone else for what happened."

Most children suffer guilt in silence. Others may show feelings of guilt by what they say or do. Children may blame themselves for everything that goes wrong, become perfectionists in all they do, or they may play out themes of blame with their toys. I have heard children tell their dolls that they were "stupid" and "dumb" and watched as they punished them for simple mistakes. I have watched as children rejected favorite stuffed animal friends and told them they didn't love them anymore. The self-esteem of every one of these children was suffering. They felt they were stupid, dumb, and unlovable. They had taken on a responsibility that did not belong to them.

One seven-old-year girl told me she felt guilty for running from the scene of a crime. Everyone thought she was running for help. She confessed to me that she was really running to get away so she wouldn't be hurt next. Another child told me he felt bad because he was glad the trauma happened to his sibling. He said, "I shouldn't feel this way, but I'm glad it wasn't me!" Many children wrestle with feelings of guilt for not being able to stop the tragedy or for not knowing "what to do."

You can help your child recognize that feelings of guilt are normal and help them in situations where they need to recognize right from wrong. Let children know that feelings of guilt happen in everyone from time to time and are a sign of healthy emotions. It is important to reassure children they are *not* responsible for another person's actions or choices.

After a near-death experience, a client told me it was a "gift" that her life had been spared. She wisely concluded that "to spend the rest of my life in guilt is a terrible waste of the gift."

Anger

To be human is to know anger. Like any emotion, there is a healthy way and an unhealthy way to act on or express it. Most people recognize there are healthy aspects to anger and that when it is expressed appropriately it can also be important to spiritual health. Even many religions and belief systems see it as a positive emotion. It can help people identify and clarify the need for change, self-care, and action. Adults and children who suppress anger often develop physical and emotional manifestations. In situations like this, anger can be toxic to the soul.

Reasons for Anger

There are as many reasons to be angry as there are people who have suffered a traumatic experience. The angry emotions that surface in the aftermath of trauma are often confusing and frightening to both children and their parents. Rage can look and feel disorganized, all-consuming, and insurmountable. By understanding some of the reasons for their feelings, you can show children how to be helped, rather than hindered, by angry emotions. Following are some common ways anger affects those who've experienced trauma:

- Most people feel angry when they've lost trust. The sudden and irrational nature of trauma contradicts the notion that the world and others around you will always behave in rational and predictable ways. Instead trauma brings a feeling of chaos and apprehension and the idea that if this could happen, *anything* could. Consequently, children lose trust in the order and security of their lives. They may resent the way everything inside them feels suddenly and dramatically changed. For most, anger is an expression of deep fears and tortured conflict.

- *Anger may result when everyone else seems to be happily going on with life despite what happened.* Children may resent the fact that after a time others don't seem to understand their continued upset. They may be angry at those who seem to have no problem feeling happy again. They may be bewildered when people greet them as if the trauma they experienced had never happened. Some children find this to be more relieving than distressing; however, pretending that nothing happened does a disservice to children. Children need to be acknowledged, if even briefly, for what they went through. Otherwise the message they sometimes hear is "It's no big deal," or "Why should I talk about it if no one else does?"

  There may be an outpouring of support in the form of cards, gifts, and special attention that is validating to kids immediately after a trauma. When people move on with their lives some children may feel as if others have stopped caring. Sometimes a child's anger stems from feelings of loneliness and hurt. When others move on they may feel left behind.

  Children may need help in understanding that the effects of trauma can be long-lasting for those who experience it and that it will be different for those who haven't been through what they have. Let kids know that just because others are able to move on doesn't mean they have stopped caring, it just means they didn't experience the trauma in the same way the children did. Help your kids recognize their anger and validate their reasons for having it.

- *Anger may be a result of loss of confidence in the judicial process and the belief that justice prevails.* Children may question their safety and express surprise when guilty offenders are not put or kept in jail for their crimes. They may not feel protected by the very systems set up for their safety.

- *People impacted by trauma rarely hear apologies from whoever or whatever caused the tragedy.* Maybe there is no one responsible for the trauma that impacted your child (e.g., if it was a natural disaster, accident, house fire). Even when there is someone to blame and hold responsible, that person may lack remorse or avoid an apology for fear it will be considered an admission of guilt. Whatever the case may be, it can be more difficult to resolve an experience without an apology.

When I was a teenager, I struggled with the fact that the two offenders who caused the car crash I was in never apologized for the pain they inflicted. Time and time again I told others, "If only they would say they were sorry. That's why I'm angry. They don't care about what they did."

Would a simple apology really have changed anything? It wouldn't have helped everything, but it would have given me back something I had lost. It may have resolved what was at the core of my rage. I didn't want justice or punishment or money. More than anything, I wanted the two people who almost took my life and the life of my friend to express regret for their actions. I wanted the assurance that they had understood what they had done and that they would never again do it to another person. I wanted to go on believing that no one would intentionally try to take another person's life. I soon learned that I would need to reconstruct some of my beliefs.

You may be finding it difficult to pick up the pieces of your beliefs as well, but in time your life can move on despite your broken ideals. Your child needs you to put the pieces back together in a way that will be helpful to them. Do this by reminding them of all that is good and constant in the world. Focus on what's right while you learn to reconcile what's wrong. Balance the tragedy with the joy.

If pain, loss, and disillusionment are all children see, that's what their life will be filled with. You can tell children that just as the anger and pain they hold is not all of who they are, neither is life only about pain and loss. Make sure that their view of life includes all there is to life besides this tragedy.

Forgiveness

Is it important to encourage children to forgive and forget? Does forgiveness need to be a part of a child's recovery process? Does forgiveness even apply to victims impacted by unspeakable crimes? Do your spiritual practices and beliefs mandate that you forgive others no matter what atrocity they have committed?

Forgiveness means different things to different people. For most, it is a very hard thing to do. It is a personal decision based on individual feelings and beliefs. Forgiveness is an issue your children are likely to face. It is a concern they might wrestle with when someone has directly been the cause of their pain and suffering. You will want to handle the issue of forgiveness with openness, based on your own beliefs and your child's feelings.

Forgiveness in general needs to be in ready supply—the ability to be a family usually depends on it. To be sure, it is sometimes easier to forgive those you love than a stranger who causes you or your children harm. But the benefits of forgiving are too important to the well-being of your child's life to ignore.

Forgiving Is Not Excusing

It is important to explain to children who have been hurt by trauma what forgiveness is and is not. You do not have to remove blame from someone who has committed an act of injustice in order to forgive them. On the contrary, these individuals must be held accountable for their actions whenever possible. If they weren't to blame, they wouldn't need forgiveness.

Forgiving Is Not Forgetting

Forgiving is remembering the experience and accepting what has happened. It may also mean remembering what was learned as a result of the traumatic event. For example, as trauma survivors, children may have learned how to grieve and how to be safer or more prepared. They may have learned who to trust, who to be cautious around, and what meaning life has for them. Children may have discovered strengths in themselves that they never knew they had.

Forgiving Is Letting Go

You and your children may be filled with resentment and bitterness because of what has happened to your family. Forgiving does not mean hearts will be free from all feelings of resentment or that you won't continue to wish for justice. But when you are consumed by hate, all you are is hate. There is no room for anything else.

Forgiveness is in everyone's own best interest. It means letting go of destructive feelings in yourself and toward others. It builds up what's good in you and let's go of what will only harm you more. Forgiving is the path to peace for you and your child. Forgiveness is part of healing the soul.

Here are a few suggestions for how to help children learn to forgive:

- Listen to and be understanding of all the reasons children might not want to forgive.

- Acknowledge that what happened will always be wrong and will never be forgotten.

- Point out what has been learned as a result of their experience.

- Look at and talk about the strengths children have shown or developed through the experience.

- Talk about the way hate can consume everything good inside of you. (Give them some examples of hateful experiences you or your child have experienced in the past.)

- Talk about the way forgiveness feels when you give it. (Give examples of times when you or your child have offered forgiveness in past situations.)

- Talk about the way forgiveness feels when you receive it. (Give examples of ways you and your child have received forgiveness in the past.)

- Ask children what they think might be good about forgiveness. Why do they think it's important?

- Share your belief, idea, or hope about what is right about forgiveness (e.g., forgiveness gets rid of hurtful feelings and replaces them with acceptance and peace).

- Acknowledge that forgiveness takes time and may not happen easily or all at once.

- Encourage children to forgive when it feels genuine and right for them. Assure them they need not feel ashamed or wrong if they feel unable to forgive. Tell them forgiving is a different process for everyone and that you will support them whether they forgive or not.

The Gift of Spiritual Support

Helping children find spiritual support in the aftermath of trauma is an important way to teach them the value of their souls. If that support comes from you, remember to share the specific beliefs and religious or cultural views you hold in a positive, nonjudging way.

If attending a place of worship is part of your family's routine, by all means maintain this practice and ask the religious leaders in your faith to address questions and concerns you and your child might be facing.

If you don't practice or maintain a spiritual foundation, your child may be asking for one. Be understanding of your child's desire to find a secure belief system. Be open to exploring this resource for yourself and your child. Spiritual development can happen at any age and is usually a lifelong process. Trauma may cause you to pay attention to it right now, but it doesn't have to end when the crisis is over.

Given something to believe in, children may never have to face a life without meaning. This may be the most important gift you could ever give your child.

Kevin's faith wasn't lost. It was challenged. In the end he told me that the sad tragedy he endured had given him more faith than he had ever felt in his life. The experience, he said, proved to him how much humans need God. He concluded that when we don't depend on beliefs for guidance through life, terrible mistakes are made. Life-and-death mistakes.

I asked Kevin to write a letter to his grandmother. I explained that, even though she had died, expressing his thoughts and feelings to her might be helpful. He wrote:

> I want you to know I'm growing up better because of you. The truth is I always loved you and I always will, and I know you knew that by all the fun times we had together. Anything else I ever said to you besides that was just plain stupid. The truth is, Grandma, you did bug me about stuff sometimes. I know I bugged you, too. But you never deserved to die the way you did. I guess I thought you would live forever, and then to have you gone because of what he did is something I will never understand. What I do understand is Grandpa needed help and I wish we could've seen it before he took your life. How did he hide it from all of us? I wish you could've told us. The people who knew didn't tell us either. They said they used to hear loud fights and screaming from your house. They said they thought they should mind their own business. Now you're gone and it's too late. I want you to know I helped raise money for victims of domestic violence and I contributed it all in memory of you. I miss you and will remember you forever.
>
> Love, Kevin

And to his grandfather he wrote:

> I will be sure to make my life different from yours and do the right thing if I ever get married. Sorry you didn't learn at seventy what I have learned at twelve. No one deserves

to go through what she did. You can't hide anymore. We know now that you hurt her and exploded a lot. You should've stopped and got help or left to protect her from the monster inside you! I know now I didn't kill Grandma with my words and God didn't make it happen either. You and you alone are responsible. It's between you and God now. Sorry you didn't learn that sooner. I have, and my faith is the most important thing I have. It's taught me what real love is supposed to be. I loved you, Granddad, but I can't honestly say I do anymore. I've accepted you're gone and that you're not who I thought you were. I hope you'll find help and be able to feel what you've really done. I can't seem to forgive you yet, but I know God understands that, too. Maybe someday you'll find forgiveness for yourself.

Kevin

As Kevin learned to face all his thoughts and feelings about what happened, he continued to be strengthened by his faith. It was not an easy road, and at times he fell into periods of deep despair. In the process, Kevin learned to grieve and express his loss in both open and private ways. This helped him explain his feelings of depression and his profound disappointment in life. Through it all he figured out a lot about his own values and what he wanted out of life.

For Kevin, searching his soul led him back to a foundation of faith and hope. From that foundation, he was able to heal.

5

Healing Through Grieving

"Someday I'll be with her again."

🐾 *Every school day Cody and his mom shared the same morning routine. She walked with him to his first grade classroom at 8:15 in the morning, and then she walked the long way home for daily exercise. After school she would wait by the fence where all the parents did and they would walk home together, each sharing the day's events. Cody liked school but he always looked forward to walking home with his mom. Cody liked to talk, and she was always happy to listen.*

Then one day the routine changed. Cody's teacher told him he needed to leave school a half hour early. She told him he was to go to the office where his father was waiting for him. He thought she sounded mad. No one had told him his dad was coming today, and he wondered why he got to leave school so soon. He thought that it might be a surprise and started to feel excited. And then he saw his dad's face.

The words he spoke to Cody came out slow and tired. Cody wondered what was wrong with his dad. He couldn't finish his sentences. What was he saying? It made no sense to him. Someone closed a door and they were in a room all alone. "Where's Mom,

Dad?" he asked. And again, Cody couldn't understand what his dad said. He was talking too slow. He wasn't making sense. He kept saying, "Mommy got hit by a car. She went to the hospital, but they couldn't save her. Mommy is gone. She died Cody."

Quietly, they both picked up his belongings and walked out the door. Grown-ups were all around saying things to his dad, but he couldn't understand their words. Cody was too busy thinking about the fence in the front of the school where other parents had started gathering to pick up their kids. Cody was sure his mom would be there. Every day she met him at the same place. "Won't Mom be here, Dad?" His dad answered slowly again, "No, Cody. Mom can't be here. Get in the car. Uncle Jim is driving us home."

That night Cody heard his mom's name on the news. He looked up to see the television screen and saw the mangled car that hit her. He thought he saw her leg laying twisted in the wreckage and her blood on the road.

Over the next several days, Cody overheard the story of his mom's death again and again. He heard all about the man who got drunk at 8:30 in the morning and crashed into his mom as she walked on the side of the road.

At the funeral Cody appeared preoccupied and detached. He didn't look sad or upset. In fact, Cody seemed bored. No one ever saw him cry. Those at the funeral were deeply distressed by his apparent lack of feelings and grief. Someone said he didn't seem to care that his mom was gone. Someone else suggested he was spoiled and selfish. Even at seven, they thought, he should be able to show respect for his mom's memory.

When he went back to school, Cody's teachers also said he appeared unaffected. As if it had never happened.

The school counselor referred Cody to my office for grief counseling. His father was willing to bring him in once, but was doubtful he really needed counseling because, as he said, "Cody wasn't in any grief." He told me Cody seemed fine. He thought Cody might be too young to really understand it all and that he was glad. Maybe it was for the best. He didn't want his son to be going through what he was. Why try to make him feel things he didn't need to?

But his father also said he wanted to be sure nothing was wrong with him. He, too, was perplexed as to why Cody never cried and why he hadn't missed his mom yet. He knew he loved her very much. They were close, and because she worked at home they were together every day. Cody's father told me, "He says he knows she's

never coming back, but he laughs like it's all a big joke. It hurts. I
get really angry at the disrespect he has for his mom. She loved him
so much. How can he act like that?"

Cody joined our session and agreed to see me without his dad.
We talked about my job and why he was seeing me. Cody told me
his mom had died. He explained that "a bad man" killed her because
he was drinking alcohol and it made him drive crazy. Cody appeared
happy, bright, and excited to play.

I asked Cody to draw me a picture of his family. He drew his
mom and dad standing together on grass near flowers. He put
himself up high in a hot-air balloon above them. Black clouds, drawn
in sharp heavy lines, covered the top of his balloon. Although the
threatening black clouds and escaping balloon indicated he was
experiencing a great deal of distress, Cody wasn't ready to see his
loss or be in reality. He was not ready to live in a world where his
mother did not exist.

Cody had a wound so deep that he tried to avoid remembering
his mom. In the months ahead, I learned what a powerful medicine
truth would be in resolving the anxieties Cody secretly struggled
with. Until the symptoms brought on by the trauma were resolved,
Cody could not express his loss or find the relief he needed through
a natural grieving process.   ෨

Loss Is Part of Trauma

There are many kinds of loss that can occur in the course of a traumatic event. Not all grief stems from death. Your child's loss may
involve a person, but it may also involve a place or belonging. Some
children lose feelings. The loss of safety, trust, routine, or sense of
security in life can significantly alter a child's worldview.

A twelve-year-old girl heard about a kidnapping and strangula-
tion of a child who lived in a different state than she did. She was
affected by the news for weeks. She told me it had "changed her." A
trauma can produce a loss of innocence about life.

Being exposed to trauma is like being exposed to a voracious
epidemic. Everyone who knows about it will be infected on some
level. Your child may have been exposed intimately or from a distance, but regardless of the way trauma made it's way into your
child's life, grief and loss are likely to follow.

If your child has been exposed to trauma or news of a trauma,
you can expect to see a wide range of reactions. Almost any emotion

or physical symptom can surface following a loss. Grief-related symptoms may show up immediately or appear many months later. Reactions often go unrecognized in children because visible signs are not always evident. Symptoms of grief in young children are more likely to show up in the form of misbehavior and angry outbursts (Krupnick 1984). This can make it more difficult for parents to respond supportively to children's grief. While the pangs of loss are likely to show up in some form, every child's experience is different.

People usually assume that children are coping better than they are because children's sadness can be so fleeting. Grief may cause young children to be quiet and sad one moment and playful and animated the next. Children often face sadness and then ignore it. Krupnick's research supports the idea that children alternately approach and avoid their feelings to avoid being overwhelmed (Krupnick 1984). Grieving is a process that will come and go for most.

Even though there are no simple answers or solutions to the pain of loss, there are many ways you can help your child through the experience of grief. First, it is important to understand how traumatic grief differs from other forms of grief you may have experienced.

A Different Kind of Grief

When grief is the result of a traumatic incident, the process of mourning becomes complicated. Grief symptoms can be delayed because of disturbing trauma symptoms, such as intrusive thoughts and images, hypervigilence, physical reactions, or anxiety. Or grieving may be incomplete because of long-term legal proceedings that continually bring the trauma back to life.

Trauma survivors often find it difficult to experience a "natural" grieving process, in part because trauma itself is so "unnatural." The grief that results from trauma must follow a different course for its resolution.

Take Care of Trauma Symptoms First

According to child researchers Robert S. Pynoos and Spencer Eth, efforts at relieving traumatic anxiety take priority over mourning (Pynoos and Eth 1985b). Children do not have the energy to grieve while they are struggling to cope with symptoms related to trauma. When distress gradually reduces and thoughts and feelings no longer frighten or worry them, children generally feel more free to mourn their losses. Successful grieving cannot take place until stress and anxiety are relieved first.

෫ෂ *Cody liked to draw as much as he liked to talk. Every week he came in excitedly to my office, made himself comfortable at my table, and began to draw everything on his mind. He told me he saved up all the "stuff" he thought about for his appointments with me. His pictures were "too scary" for his family and sometimes they got mad when he drew "blood and guts." That week I asked him to draw me a picture of what happened to his mom. He worried it might make me mad the way it had his grandmother. I assured Cody that he could draw anything and it would not upset me.*

Through his art, Cody showed me the disturbing images he saw in his mind every time he thought about his mother. Cody drew a picture of what he believed had happened to his mom, based on the television news report, parts of conversations he'd heard, and what he believed to be true. In his picture his mom's body was splattered in pieces across the road and her blood was everywhere. This graphic image shot through his mind with any reminder of her, so he quickly learned how to forget about her memory by distracting himself. It was a lot of work and effort with limited results. It made it impossible for Cody to grieve his mom's death.

It's hard to say how long Cody could have carried the frightening images that made mourning impossible. Perhaps a lifetime. At age seven, Cody had the opportunity to resolve these troublesome symptoms so that he could continue his development without their influence and benefit from the ultimate healing which the grief process provides.

In this case the truth helped Cody more than anything else. His mom had died of internal injuries, and contrary to his mental pictures, her body had remained intact. I was able to correct his misinformation and show him the written police report which supported my information. Cody's face showed his relief. Discovering this truth provided the opening I needed to help Cody learn how to cope with these and other symptoms.

In a period of several months in weekly counseling, Cody learned to successfully express, understand, and manage the scary pictures in his mind. He was finally free to remember his mother. The troubling images stopped and nightmares, which he'd also kept secret, went away. Soon he began to openly talk about his mom, and his grief could finally be expressed.

Symptoms of post-traumatic stress can be so disturbing and painful that people will go to great lengths to ignore them or cover them up. It's not uncommon for adolescents and adults to begin self-medicating their pain with drugs or alcohol. Younger children numb themselves through whatever behaviors work for them. Before your child can grieve the losses inherent in any tragedy, it is crucial that traumatic symptoms such as Cody's be addressed first.   ✒

Losing Someone Close

When children lose a close loved one through trauma they may be totally consumed by symptoms of stress and fear or totally lost in denial. Either way, children will need an unlimited supply of patience and understanding as they struggle to believe what still may feel unreal. Life irrevocably changes when a loved one dies. Like adults, children must grapple with the new reality.

What You Can Say

Your child may ask difficult questions about death and about why the trauma happened. You will not always know the "right" thing to say. No one ever has all the right answers to a child's questions and concerns. The best place to start is with the simple truth. The following are some suggestions of things you can say to your child's questions:

- Death is a physical reality that happens to every living thing. The body stops working and cannot come back.

- People can die at any age.

- Most of the time, people who are sick or injured get better. People who are taken to the hospital do not always die. They go to hospitals to help them get well.

- Even though most people are good and know how to do the right things, some people aren't and they do things that hurt others.

- There are still people you can trust to do the right things. (Make a list: for example, police, rescue workers, friends, relatives, etc.)

- Most people who get hurt can get better. Sometimes they get hurt so bad, they can't get better.

- You are not to blame.

- Your loved one did not die because they wanted to leave you.

- Death is permanent and sad.

- You won't always feel as sad as you do today.

- In time, the happy memories you have of your loved one will replace the sad memories you have now.

Explain the Language of Death

Words can create confusion for kids already perplexed by the events around them. Clarify the meaning of words and rituals such as: wake, passed away, expired, casket, visitation, hearse, memorial, celebration of life, candlelight vigil, grave, burial, widow/widower, headstone, cremation, ashes, urn, etc. When you explain the language, you teach children how to understand a part of death. This helps them successfully join others in mourning.

Like adults, children can find comfort when people come together in their grief. Make sure your child can understand enough to feel included in what's happening around them.

When Loss Is the Result of Homicide

Researchers acknowledge that homicide creates a different kind of grief because of the rage it evokes. Grief is prolonged and complicated for family and friends of a homicide victim (Allen 1980). The knowledge of how the victim was killed and the lack of dignity he or she suffered are difficult images to live with. Intense feelings of anger, blame, and repulsion are often directed toward the perpetrator.

Often the criminal justice system slows down the grieving process when closure around a case is not made or appears to be made unjustly. Children may need your help as they struggle to understand the act of murder and the intentional taking of a human life.

Children may experience strong feelings of revenge. Though revenge fantasies may slow down the grief process even further, they are necessary and important reactions for children to express. Expect to see them and learn to accept them. Children will need your continued support and understanding as the legal case unfolds.

Grieving Natural Disaster, Suicide, Family Violence, and Hate Crimes

Natural Disaster

Every year natural disasters touch the lives of thousands of people. When nature's fury is unleashed, floods, hurricanes, fires, earthquakes, and tornadoes threaten everything in its path. Even when lives seem to be miraculously spared, families have much to grieve.

The losses are staggering. Homes, businesses, income, property, furnishings, family keepsakes, and cherished belongings are just a few examples. If your family has survived a natural disaster you know only too well all the ongoing ways your life has been disrupted. The process of repairing and rebuilding a life that once was prolongs the stress and sadness you feel. The physical and emotional tasks that need to be completed may feel endless.

Victims of disaster often say they feel like life will never be the same, and they are probably right. It can feel like a whole new world must be reconstructed. This is difficult to do when your children need you perhaps more than ever before, though you need to begin putting the pieces of your family's life back together again.

Trauma isn't over just because it stops. A ten-year-old boy whose home was the victim to a forest fire told me, "I just don't feel like I use to. The fire burned me down inside just like it did our house."

He continued to feel the effects of his loss, lingering like the smoldering ashes in the canyons surrounding the land where his home use to stand. As with any traumatic event, the effects are far-reaching. When the world of nature becomes such a destructive force that it overpowers a child's physical surroundings, and the adults they trust can't do anything to stop it, all security goes up in smoke.

It's natural for children to form a bond of attachment to an inanimate object. The need for attachment is so strong that it is helpful when children have favorite objects to help comfort them. Children may be especially upset if they lost a favorite sweater, toy, book, blanket, necklace, doll, or teddy bear. The loss of these possessions are the loss of sacred parts of themselves. Inherent in these lost belongings lies the threat of death. If a toy can be destroyed, so can you. And so can they. Perhaps for the first time, death may feel real.

Children have reason to be anxious and reason to need you. The lack of warning, dramatic changes caused by the devastation, duration and degree of the threat, and lack of shelter and financial worries may be some of the difficult factors that will impact your child's recovery.

Emotional First Aid

The most important tool in your first-aid kit is you. Children are remarkably resilient when they need to be, and when the adults around them build up their security they can learn to be strong survivors. Love your child in all the ways outlined in this book and your child can learn to grow through this experience.

Be honest with children about what is happening and what has happened. Here are some suggestions of what you might say to offer reassurance:

- This is really hard for everyone right now. Lots of people want to help us.

- We're doing everything we can to get things back to normal. It will take some time.

- You can keep a bag of your special belongings right next to the door so we can take them with us if we need to leave again.

- We are safe now, and we'll continue to do whatever will help us stay safe and protected.

- You are my most valuable "belonging." Nothing else matters to me the way you do. I am grateful we have each other.

Suicide

Hearing about suicide or knowing someone who has taken their own life is frightening to children. When the child loses a loved one to suicide, grieving is complicated by anger, confusion, guilt, and the traumatic images of the way the deceased person took his or her life.

The knowledge that suicide is even a choice can be disturbing information. Children may never have imagined or considered the possibility before. It may plant seeds of doubt concerning their own impulse control and capacity to kill themselves. Here are some of the common questions children wonder about:

- How do you kill yourself?

- Why would you do that?

- What makes people want to do it?

- What did it look like?

- Could the same thing happen to me?

- Why couldn't someone stop it?

- What would it feel like?

I remember hearing a tragic story in the news when I was a young girl. A child had died after he purposely suffocated himself with a plastic bag. I soon began paying special attention to the plastic bags from the dry cleaners that I found in various closets in our home. I noticed they had warnings written on them, printed in bold red letters that read: "Danger! Keep out of reach of children! Suffocation may result!"

For a period of time after that, I felt nervous being in the same room with a plastic bag. I worried that "it would get me," and that somehow one might blow over my head and do me in. Like most children who hear about such tragedies, I wasn't able to comprehend the act of suicide or let go of the anxiety it generated in me. Adults need to make sure children understand how things happen. It will be important for your child to talk about the ways suicide has impacted them.

It is equally important to address the questions and concerns your child may have around the choice of suicide. When discussing it, be direct and firm when you say, suicide is the wrong choice.

What you can say *about suicide*:

- There are other options every person can take. People who have committed suicide didn't know or believe in other options. They lost hope and didn't know how to get it back.

- The truth is we all experience times of hopelessness in our lives. We need to share those feelings right away with people who understand.

- No matter how much you love someone, you can't always save them. It's never anyone else's fault.

Reassure children that you will help protect and guide them through their own times of hopelessness. Some things that you can say to convey this are:

- I will always be here to listen and help you with scary thoughts and feelings.

- We can always find solutions to your problems, no matter how impossible you might think it is at the time.

- Nothing you feel or think about could ever stop me from loving you.

- There is nothing you can't tell me.

- There is nothing I won't help you with.

- It's okay to talk to someone else if you need to. I will help you find someone different than me to talk to if you'd like.

- Using drugs and alcohol to feel better will only makes things worse. It can be tempting because in the beginning you can be fooled into thinking it helps you. Drugs and alcohol eventually take your hope away. They drain you of what's good and positive in yourself. The easiest way to feel better is to directly face whatever you are bothered by.

When Children Consider Suicide

A trauma may impact children to such a degree that they think about wanting to die or actually attempt to hurt or kill themselves. Thoughts of suicide are serious at any age and require immediate professional intervention.

Feelings of hopelessness and engaging in unsafe or risk-taking behaviors are only a few of the symptoms you might see. It is important that you find a professional counselor who can help identify and assess your child's risk factors. Without treatment, your child may face dangerous short-term and long-term consequences. Taking your child to a counselor or therapist can help counteract the sense of helplessness your child may feel.

In some children suicidal thoughts and feelings are an attempt to understand or make sense of death. After jumping from a jungle gym in what he said was an attempt to "kill" himself, one nine-year-old told me, "When I did it, I never thought I'd get a black-and-blue knee! That hurt! I just wanted to see where my uncle went so I could tell my mom and dad." Regardless of the true intention of a child's comments or actions, these situations need to be evaluated and assessed by a professional who has experience working with children.

The recognition that your child would consider taking his or her own life is both terrifying and difficult to comprehend. Most parents would rather convince themselves it could never really happen. They are eager to believe that their child is just going through "another stage" or is too young to really be at risk. Don't fall into this trap of denial.

To find out if your child has thoughts or ideas of self-harm, ask him or her directly. Take all statements and behaviors seriously. Even if your child denies thoughts of suicide, get help at once if your child's attitude or behaviors worry you. Any doubt or concern you have about your child's safety or state of mind is reason enough to seek help.

Family Violence

Children who have witnessed domestic violence in their homes are in special need of professional help. Many have been exposed to repeated and ongoing acts of trauma and loss. Growing up in a chronic state of fear affects a child's ability to grow and develop in natural ways. Many have learned to accommodate unusual physical symptoms and reactions because they have had no other choice.

When a person is abusive to their partner, they cannot be a good parent. With every physical, emotional, spiritual, or psychological blow, children are learning inaccurate and dangerous messages. When women are the object of men's tyranny, the developing attitudes and self-esteem of boys and girls who witness it is adversely affected. Most will view violence as a "normal" way of life. It is not uncommon for these children to bury years of grief. Professional counseling can help children understand and identify the many losses they sustained and help teach them ways to grieve.

Professional intervention is necessary for all child victims of domestic violence. Research is showing that observing violence in the family causes developmental damage to children and left untreated, children who witness violence may be at a higher risk of perpetrating acts of violence against others in the future (Jaffe, Wilson, and Wolfe 1986). They often enter young adulthood with the enormous weight of unresolved grief upon them. They may also carry attitudes and values that perpetuate disrespect and inequity between people because of what they experienced themselves.

These attitudes must be addressed. Children need to learn that value and self-worth are not dependent on gender or on the ability to have power over others. A healthy balance of both feminine and masculine traits will strengthen your children's resiliency and their safety in relationships.

A counselor can help steer your children away from violence against another person's heart, mind, body, or soul. Counseling can help children resolve the trauma of domestic violence, grieve the inherent losses, and learn to grow healthy relationships.

Hate Crimes

Race, religion, gender, sexual orientation, profession, and other personal characteristics are sometimes the focal point for acts of human cruelty, rage, and even murder. When hate results in crime, communities are hurt, families suffer, and children are confused and frightened.

Victims of hate suffer many losses. Children lose confidence in the world when they have been directly or indirectly impacted by a hate crime. The grieving process is complicated by anger and fear.

Like other emotions, hate has the potential of undermining the emotional, physical, and spiritual health of a person. A twelve-year-old girl told me hate can be like a sliver imbedded under the skin. It can be hard to get at, it hurts every time you move or touch anything, and if you don't get it out, it can get infected and become a bigger problem.

Without help, hate can become dangerously embedded like a sliver in the soul. Children who have been directly or indirectly impacted may need help in resolving senseless acts of revenge, allowing them to process the grief that follows and avoid becoming obsessed with reciprocal hate of the perpetrator.

Adults have an obligation to help children develop an intolerance for hate crimes, empathy for victims, and respect for human differences. Whether they are the victim of a playground bully or a racist terrorist, children need to know what actions and attitudes to take to help extinguish the flames of hatred.

The following story is for young children impacted by hate crimes. "It Happened Out of Hate" was written to help children express their own experiences and to better understand the experiences of others impacted by this crime. It is one tool you can use to help children move through the process of grieving and help instill the value of love and understanding for all people.

"It Happened Out of Hate"— A Story for Children

Following is a story about a child impacted by a hate crime and how she or he felt after it happened. Your child can add to the story by completing the exercises in italics inside the story.

&ea *Someone in my family got hurt. Just for being different. It happened out of hate.*

I hate bee stings, I hate cleaning my room, I hate going places I don't think will be fun. And I hate what those people did to hurt my family. It hurts to hate.

What happened to someone you know: (Draw and color a picture).

I feel mad. I'm tired of always being different. I want my family to change.

What's different about your family: (Draw and color a picture). What's different about you: (Draw and color a picture).

I worry that someone in my family will get hurt again, while they're going to work, going to the store, going to school, going out to jog. I don't think we're safe anywhere anymore.

I feel afraid. How could someone hate us if they didn't even know us? It's not fair. I want to move and hide.

I have a counselor. She said I was right, what happened to us wasn't fair. I asked her why some people are mean to people like my family member. She said some people hate because they are afraid of what's different, and that some people might act mean in ways that others have been mean to them. She said when people use their hate to hurt others it is wrong. She said what happened to my family was a crime.

I never knew it was against the law to hate. She told me feelings are never against the law, but how our feelings make us act might be. She believes no matter why, and whatever the reason, hurting people is never okay.

My counselor said hate takes up all the room inside us when it happens. She said hate changes the way we think, the way we act, and the things we say.

I learned that hate changes the way we see through our eyes, the way we hear when we listen, the way we sound when we talk. And that everyone feels it sometimes.

Your feelings of hate happen when: (Draw and color a picture).

I thought grown-ups knew how to be nice. The grown-ups who did this scared me. My counselor said most people have learned how to respect everyone, no matter who they are. That means they treat all people in kind ways. My counselor asked me to think about all the grown-ups I like and feel safe with.

Grown-ups you feel safe with: (Draw and color a picture). You can tell when someone doesn't like me when: (Draw and color a picture).

My counselor said everything different about me makes me special. How I think, feel, act, look, and sound. We are who we are. Some days I still don't like being different. Other days I'm happy being exactly who I am. My counselor said most people feel that way no matter who they are. I found out that even if one person learns from me that being different is okay it will plant a seed. And I learned that love can grow anywhere.

What you like about being different: (Draw and color a picture).

I know now we can't change every wrong thing that happens to us. And I understand why it's never okay to tease or use words that hurt people who are different.
  When we see a rainbow, watch fireworks, hold a puppy, taste our favorite ice cream, open a present, hear our favorite song, smell home-baked bread, we aren't so different.
  I'm learning how to plant the seeds of love and understanding.

How you might plant the seeds of love and understanding: (Draw and color a picture).

Let Your Child Grieve

Grieving can be hard work. Expressing the pain of loss can be tiring and draining. But unless the work is done, open wounds can never heal, and your child will not have the opportunity to feel whole again.

Sometimes the only way to release the deepest parts of yourself, buried by pain, is through tears. Let your child cry. Help your child understand that crying is healthy. Tears have even been found to contain certain chemicals that are natural pain relievers. They cleanse the heart, mind, body, and soul by relieving stress.

After a a devastating experience, it's difficult, as well as counterproductive to "put on a happy face." Let children feel their hurt. Don't try to talk them out of their grief or tone down their reactions. Sadness deserves a place in your child's life, unhidden and undisguised.

If you have a hard time expressing your own sadness or tend to hide your feelings to "protect" others, it will require special effort on your part to let your child learn how to let grieving happen. Some children will need simple companionship without pressure to talk or do anything. Don't rush children into the grieving process and don't be in a hurry to get them through it. Tell children they can take all the time they need. Learn to be with them in their pain without trying to change their experience. By doing this, you can teach children the importance of mourning in healthy ways.

Healing Tools: Activities, Rituals, and Pets

Activities Help Children Grieve Their Loss

When you participate with children in meaningful activities surrounding the trauma they experienced, it is a way for you to begin sharing their loss.

Find activities that will provide you with opportunities to talk about who and what your child has lost. During these times you can also talk about ways the trauma impacted you. Tell them about your own unique experience and perspectives to help children identify theirs. The following are suggested activities to help you begin:

- Put together a special photo album, scrapbook, or memory book, or co-write a journal or letter that talks about the life of the person lost or remembers the special memories your child has around what he or she lost.

- Create a picture collage about the person who died or around any aspect of a loss.

- Write a poem, prayer, or eulogy about what happened. Writing letters to the deceased can also be healthy and healing. If your children would like anything they've written to be read aloud to family and/or friends, arrange a time to do that.

- Make a display about the loss. A public display of the community's grief can be a powerful healing tool. Some people may be offended by "shrines" constructed in the memory of a person or event, but many others find honor in such displays. If such an idea is desired by the children, then support it. Others who may be offended should be respected and supported in their choice not to participate. In the same way some children will be eager to take such displays down after a certain time, others will want them up permanently to never forget or deny the event. Both needs are real and valuable. Let children decide.

- Plan a celebration to remember what the person or loss meant to you.

- Plant a memorial tree or flower in remembrance.

- Make a donation or contribution to a special cause in memory of your loss.

- Join community activities that are organized around the same or similar loss as yours.

- Join a family support group or offer your child the opportunity to be part of a children's support group. Sometimes children interact much easier with their peers than with adults. They need to know they are not alone or "different" because of what happened to them.

- With children's permission, tape-record or write down their memories of who or what they lost and give it to them as a gift in the future. Young children are especially grateful for this when they are older. Special memories can remain vivid and intact with your help.

- Playing new and familiar board games may provide the opportunity for relaxed discussions.

- Remember to tell children how valuable it is to hear and share their memories and loss. Be creative and come up with an activity that is inspired by your child.

Rituals Can Help Children Grieve

Special services can help children learn to grieve in both private and public ways. Adults may assume that a child does not need to attend the funeral or memorial service of someone they lost. When my daughter was four, her grandmother expressed concern that I was bringing her to a friend's funeral. She thought she was too young and worried that she'd be frightened or upset by it.

I explained to my daughter in detail what would happen at the service and why we were going. I told her people would be crying and sad because we would all miss Ada. I told her funerals were a special time to remember and say good-bye to someone we loved. I explained how Ada's body would be buried in the ground, and that her feelings were already gone. I told her she could come with us or stay home and play with her favorite baby-sitter. She looked at me in disbelief and said, "I loved Ada, too! Why would everyone go except me?!"

A half hour before we left, my daughter asked me for scissors and a piece of foil. She asked if I would help her cut a big red rose off our bush. She told me, "Ada loved the roses I used to bring her when I visited her. I want her to have one buried with her when I say good-bye."

At the burial, my daughter carefully stepped forward and gently placed her rose on Ada's casket. She returned and held my hand as we all said good-bye. Six years later my daughter wrote a vivid account of this memory for a homework assignment. Her participation in the grieving process had clearly impacted her in ways I had not seen. It was a positive and loving lesson about death.

Give children the option to either attend a memorial service or stay with someone they care about. After you have prepared them for everything that will happen and why, if children have the desire to be a part of the service they should be allowed to attend. If they do attend, let them be involved. Children often express the desire to participate in services by reading poems, meaningful passages, or personal writings.

Some children could care less about attending services because they aren't able to grasp the importance of such a ritual. Others will feel relieved not to go because the idea makes them feel nervous and afraid. Children who choose to stay home should be supported in making the decision they feel most comfortable with.

Pets Can Comfort

There are many benefits to having a loving pet in your home. Studies have shown that the companionship of an affectionate pet can reduce blood pressure and have a calming effect on people. After a loss, the love from an animal can provide a great deal of comfort to a child.

Cody's father tried to bring a puppy into Cody's life in the months following his mother's funeral. Cody resisted the idea initially, feeling it "would be too hard to try and love anything new." His father persisted and Cody reluctantly gave in. It was the new puppy's enthusiastic expression of unconditional love for Cody that eventually helped him make room for more love again. The puppy became a new beloved member of the family.

A pet can bring relief to a child in a way other people around them cannot. Pets can provide a sense of safety to the home and give love and companionship without demanding anything in return. Pets can comfort a child. Best of all, they bring relief to children who do not want to talk or listen to another word about the trauma they suffered. A pet isn't the answer for everyone, but it's worth considering if your child could benefit from more support. In Cody's case, his father benefited, too.

Finding Your Way to Professional Help

Seeking professional help is an important step in making a commitment to helping your children process their experience. While there are no pills or quick fixes that will enable your child to recover quickly from trauma, counseling can help alleviate suffering and provide care. Even with professional help, the emotional repair process will still happen in stages and at its own pace.

The Benefits of Counseling

You don't have to wait to see obvious signs of distress before you have a counselor intervene with your child and family. One of the greatest benefits of seeking therapeutic help is that trained trauma counselors can use techniques to help children discuss the tragedy they endured. Skilled clinicians will be able to do this in a way that will help children express the horror of their experience without becoming overwhelmed. They can provide children with the emotional support they need to recall the important details of their experience so that their loss can be grieved.

Children who receive professional help often find that counseling is a safe place where they can comfortably express their feelings of grief and loss. It can be helpful for kids to engage in play with a therapist who is specially trained to help them work through the effects of trauma. This ensures that children have ample opportunity to express their true thoughts and the full range of emotions the trauma has awakened in them.

Violent events may bring to light painful feelings from past experiences that were never addressed or that remain unresolved, like a divorce, death, or sexual abuse in a child's life. Professional intervention can ensure that these issues are properly addressed as well.

It's not uncommon for parents to be physically and emotionally less available to their children following a trauma that has impacted the whole family. You may be dealing with your own grief. Since it happened, the trauma may have temporarily changed your home routines and even your personality. Children may experience this as another loss and grieve for the way you or your home "used to be."

A counselor can help by serving as a special advocate for your child when you can't be as available to them as you would like. You deserve all the support and assistance you can get in order to be the best parent you can be through this incredibly difficult time.

The fact is, some kids just need extra help. They need professional care and attention. This does not mean your child is "crazy" or "defective." What happened was crazy; your child is not. Your child is simply responding in a normal way to an abnormal event. Your child deserves the help you can provide in the same way he or she deserves appropriate medical care when an illness cannot be treated by you or home remedies alone.

I told Cody's father he had done the right thing in bringing his son in for counseling. I explained that even though Cody didn't appear affected, his father's concern about why Cody didn't seem to care was valid. There was nothing "wrong" with Cody for needing help. The trauma of his mom's death had merely impacted him in ways we could not understand yet. In order to help Cody at this juncture in his life, we needed the time to gain both an understanding and appreciation for his initial responses. Fortunately, Cody's father gave his son that gift of time and attention.

Making the Decision

When possible, children benefit from being included in the decision-making process when making the choice to seek outside help. You may have already offered your child the opportunity to see a counselor and perhaps he or she declined, didn't care, or didn't respond to the idea. Not all children will want to open up to a stranger or like the idea of going to talk to a professional counselor.

As a responsible parent you will need to decide what is in the best interest of your child. Seeking professional help may be a decision only you can make. It is important to involve children and hear about their ideas and wishes, but be careful not to let them make the decision for you. A child of any age cannot always be expected to know what help he or she needs.

If the level of distress you and your child are experiencing is overwhelming or causing suffering which cannot be alleviated, don't delay. You and your child don't need to suffer alone. It is time to seek support when feelings of hopelessness weigh too heavy on the heart.

Choosing the Right Professional

Seek out a caring child therapist who has special training in trauma work. Child psychiatrists, clinical social workers, child psychologists, and child and family counselors may be appropriate resources. Choose someone who will consult with you first and answer any questions you may have. Most importantly, trust your feelings about whether or not this is someone you feel will care for your child in a loving and respectful manner. Your nurse practitioner or family doctor may be a good resource to call for referrals.

Prepare Your Child in Advance

You can prepare children for the experience of counseling and help them see the decision as a positive one. Following are a few examples of what you might say to prepare your child:

- You deserve special help after all you've been through.

- There are people who know what to do for you right now, and they will help you learn how to live with what happened.

- Specially trained people know and understand what you've been through and they want to help.

- It's okay not to like it, but we need to go anyway.

- I love you so much that I will do whatever it takes to help you feel better again.

- Going to a counselor can help you heal.

Letting Go

Placing your child in the hands of another adult, allowing them to care for deep personal wounds, may cause you to feel tremendous loss and inadequacy. Even when the adult is a professional helper, it can feel like a tough decision.

Perhaps until now you've been all your child has needed. You were the only one who could soothe, comfort, and "make the hurt go away." You may feel as though you are being replaced or that somehow you have failed to meet your child's deepest needs.

You will meet your child's needs when you are able to let go and do what is best for them. You will never be replaced. Letting go and asking for help is an opportunity to show your child the value in asking for help. It is an opportunity to teach your child the wisdom in recognizing and accepting your own limitations.

Your children need you to be their parent. Focus on that role. Try letting another loving and concerned adult help you in a professional capacity.

The truth is, your child's resiliency and self-confidence can grow and strengthen apart from you. Don't deny your child this experience. Your relationship will grow stronger for it. Seeking help for your child and yourself is an act of love and strength.

Stronger with Every Loss

Buried grief won't go away, but it can *get in the way*. Emotions can be frightening, but once your child's grief is recognized and expressed, the process of grieving can be healing.

After children have suffered a difficult loss, it may be hard for them to risk being close to others. It may be a challenge for children to live life without the intense fear of losing someone or something again. But with every loss, your children can grow stronger.

If you have grieved successfully in the past, you have access to more skills and knowledge to help you the next time through. It may not be any easier, but you may be able to cope in more helpful ways. Even the recognition that you will recover and find your balance again can give you the strength to move through the process of grieving. There seems to be a domino effect to loss: each experience prepares you for the next. If children are given the opportunity to successfully grieve, they will be strengthened in this way, too.

Trust in the process and prepare your child for the time it will take to heal. It can be a slow road to acceptance and peace. With your help your child can complete the journey.

Once again, Cody shared his innermost thoughts and feelings with me through his art. In the final step before grieving his loss, he expressed his feelings of rage and resentment toward the offender for taking his mom away from him. Cody drew pictures that graphically illustrated the ways he wanted to "get even." He took power and control away from that man and put it back into his own life. In time, his anger was replaced with feelings of sadness.

Cody chose to tell me about his mom's funeral by drawing a picture of it. The details of the memory he had of that day proved that the "distracted," "bored," and "uncaring" little boy everyone else thought was there was not only paying attention, but was deeply impacted.

Cody drew all of his mom's loved ones in a row. He counted every teardrop he placed on their faces. He drew halo's over their heads because, he said, "They are all good people who loved her and will miss her almost as much as me. But I'll miss her the most. She was my only mom."

Cody also drew his mom's body laying down and began a picture showing her buried in the ground. But before he finished, he quickly crossed it out. He then drew her up in the sky above everyone. He carefully put a golden halo atop her head, a big smile on her face, and gave her large wings. Cody told me in words I will never forget,

"Her body's in the ground, but she's an angel in heaven now. And I know she's happy. I can't see her, but someday I'll be with her again. I know she can watch me whenever she wants. I'm glad she's so happy!" And with a smile on his face and peace in his heart, he said, "I don't know when, but I know I'll be with her again."

6

Healing Through Humor

"Okay, so it's not as contagious as I thought."

Lisset's health seemed to be compromised following the break-in of her home. She contracted colds and fevers and complained more often of headaches. Her immune system had definitely lost the strength and resistance it once had. Despite the fact she was ill more, Lisset told me her father worried about her too much. She said he "made a big deal" every time she sneezed or looked tired. She told me that every time her dad acted like he was giving her a hug, he was really pressing his cheek against her forehead to check her temperature. "I guess he's afraid he'll miss the symptoms of a deadly plague and I'll drop dead!" Lisset rolled her eyes before she told me the results of their latest "medical emergency." She told me the only good thing about it was that her dad had been "cured" of his problem.

Lisset's dad laughed and Lisset encouraged him to tell me the story. It was the first time they had joked and kidded each other during one of our counseling sessions since they had started. As her father retold the story, my office was soon overflowing with laughter.

After school one afternoon, Lisset's father made an urgent appointment and rushed his daughter to the doctor. It was flu season and the office was bursting at the seams. They kindly squeezed her in after he described to them what Lisset had "contracted." He believed she had the beginnings of an infectious and contagious skin disease on her chin. Other cases were being reported at her school, and he was determined to nip it in the bud.

Lisset's dad told me he anticipated she would be examined under bright lights with a magnifying glass, cotton swab, surgical gloves, a skin culture, a cotton ball drenched in alcohol—something, anything, that resembled a medical procedure. Instead, the doctor used an unprotected finger to tilt Lisset's chin to one side, gave it a quick glance, closed the patient chart, and sat down. He looked at him long and hard.

The diagnosis? A pimple on top of a freckle. "For that," her dad told me, "I paid money and got labeled the 'hypochondriac parent of the month.'"

He said Lisset was so amused she couldn't even look at him. They were both unable to have eye contact until they were far away from the medical staff. They attempted to leave the office with some dignity, even though a nursing assistant yelled Stacy's "diagnosis" across the front desk as if it were a "ham on rye." They opened the door to make their escape, and Lisset's dad choked out a half-hearted cough and tried to look as sick as possible at the front of the waiting room full of desperately ill people who'd had to wait longer because of them.

They got in the car, rolled up the windows, and sat in the parking lot laughing "as hard as one humanly can." Lisset said, "It was a freckle, Dad! They thought you were so wacky! You rushed me to the doctor for a freckle!"

"Okay," he replied, "so it's not as contagious as I thought."

Lisset's dad was able to stop hovering over her and didn't focus on Lisset's health as much after that. When he began looking worried, Lisset had only to remind him of their last visit to the doctor. Lisset concluded, "At least it made us laugh again, and my dad stopped being so goofy and worried all the time."

By now you may be feeling the impact of the stories you have read throughout this book. Reading about trauma is distressing in itself, but when it has an impact on the lives of children like your own or circumstances similar to yours it is especially difficult to digest. This chapter will be different. It's about letting yourself laugh again.

Good Humor Is Goodness and Wisdom Combined

Humor is one of the most important actions you can take to heal from a stressful event. It's good "medicine" for the heart, mind, body, and soul.

Humor can begin to balance the place pain holds in your life. You can use it to ease pain and bring relief. Your child may need your help in order to put life back in balance. Laughter is a simple way to counterbalance pain. It is a wonderful tool, readily available to all.

What is "healthy" humor? The fortune cookie my daughter cracked open one night said it best: "Good humor is goodness and wisdom combined." Humor is healthy when it builds children up and expands their view of the world. It is healthy when it does not exploit anyone. Humor is not healing when it is vengeful, sarcastic, dangerous, unkind, or coerced. Healthy humor is good and wise.

Humor Can Be a Companion to Pain

You can use humor without discounting the pain and the seriousness of what has happened. Pain and humor don't have to be in opposition to each other. One does not need to be absent in order for the other to exist. Humor can be a companion to pain when it's balanced with respect and love.

Some things may be funny to your child that aren't funny to you. Just because you can't "see" what your child sees as funny, don't take away or discount his or her perspective on a situation.

If your children's humor is unkind, cruel, or offensive, talk about it with them. Sometimes in the aftermath of trauma, humor can be a feeble attempt at warding off fear or hiding true thoughts and feelings.

A sense of humor provides relief and distraction. When humor returns after a long stretch of emotional or physical suffering, it brings momentary relief of pain. Life for an instant can feel more ordinary again. Even a *taste* of the "ordinary" can feel like a feast to those starving for relief.

Can you recall times when waves of laughter "disabled" you or your child? The best memories are often those that have caused children or the adults around them to be in particularly silly situations or predicaments. Most children are especially pleased and entertained to watch their parents make "fools" of themselves.

When a sense of humor takes over, somber moods brighten and personalities unwind. In the right mood, even the ordinary day-to-day routines of life can be surprisingly entertaining. An otherwise gloomy day might transform into high comic drama. When this happens children can be immediately distracted from everything else. It's okay to encourage kids to "self-medicate" with humor and laughter. It's safe and effective.

Don't Force Humor

Sometimes people who have difficulty expressing their own sadness or pain aren't comfortable seeing anybody else's either. They may feel compelled to try and make others laugh and "put on a happy face." Trying to make children laugh when they don't want to often results in the opposite effect. Children usually grow unhappy when the fear of not being taken seriously and the shame around being ridiculed force their pain to go underground. This can lead to feelings of depression.

In families where there is an openness to emotion, children can learn to see humor in situations and learn to laugh at themselves with others. Even in the midst of tragedy, humor can be expressed in healthy ways.

Humor in the Midst of Trauma

We were driving in a desolate part of town when my friend and I were hit by the drunk driver I've referred to in previous chapters. I feared we would not be discovered in time to survive our injuries. It was unlikely that anyone had heard the crash, and we were not visible from any main roads.

I had a flash of humor that probably helped prevent panic from setting in. I saw myself dramatically crawling across land to reach help, stopping now and then to collapse in the dirt, not unlike the scene in *Gone with the Wind* when Scarlett O'Hara desperately pulled up a carrot out of the ground. I imagined newspaper headlines reading, "Teen Crawled Ten Miles: Died Two Feet from Phone Booth, Dime and Carrot in Hand." I had to laugh. Humor came through for me. It was one of my first coping mechanisms.

Remembering More Than Pain

It will be impossible to find humor in every situation. It can't always exist in the midst of horrendous acts or atrocities, but in time you will be able to remember more than just memories of the trauma. If you can share memories of times in the past that brought your children happiness, they will be encouraged to remember more than just memories of trauma. Humorous memories can remind children how to have fun again. Let your children know it's okay to remember more than pain.

For most readers, the kind of humor addressed in this chapter will probably appear down the path, far away from the tragedy and in the midst of day-to-day life once normal routines take hold again.

Stories of Humor and Healing

In the aftermath of trauma, some funny things can happen that can lighten up the healing process now and then. Most people recall the first time they were able to laugh again after a trauma. It's like rediscovering a favorite part of themselves they thought had disappeared forever.

The following anecdotes are experiences children have shared with me, and one is an experience I shared with my daughter. You may not find each of these stories amusing because humor is different for everyone. The most important thing to keep in mind as you read these stories is what the children gained by finding themselves in humorous situations again. The experiences impacted their healing process and family relationships, significantly changing their present state of mind, if even for a short while.

The parents in these stories have told me they will always appreciate the memories of these events for what they gave their children—the chance to laugh again. Through the difficult days in their healing process, they discovered there *was* joy after trauma, and it did help balance the pain. Following these events, they were able to believe and feel confident that there would be more joy in store for them in the future. Laughter helped them recover their reason for hope and optimism.

"Baggy Ankles"

&ep *It had been weeks since Stacy and her mom had gone anywhere fun together. Since the restaurant shooting, Stacy found it difficult to be around people and had little energy to socialize.*

Stacy's mother suggested they might want to attend the ballet with free tickets she had picked up at her work. It would be good, she thought, if the two of them made an effort to get out in public again. Stacy agreed to go after her mom said they could sit at the back of the performing arts center. Stacy wanted to know it would be easy to excuse herself if she began feeling faint and dizzy or if they decided they wanted to leave early.

That evening, as they dressed for the ballet, Stacy's mother discovered that all of her panty hose had runs in them. She was forced to wear knee-high stockings under her black velvet skirt which fortunately hung low enough to disguise them. The "stocking crisis" delayed them and they left later than they planned.

When they arrived at the theater, most people were already seated. As they searched for their seats, the house lights flashed and bells rang to signal that the performance was about to begin. They discovered that their seats might be located on the bottom level toward the front. Stacy's hands got sweaty and her stomach grew queasy. She didn't like the idea of sitting up close to the stage, because it made her feel "trapped" at the front. If something bad were to happen, she wanted to know she could successfully escape again.

Stacy and her mother continued to walk tentatively down the aisle toward the stage, assuming there must be a mistake. Except for a stray cough or two, a hushed silence fell over the audience. Without warning, as they approached the front-row seats, the knee-high stockings Stacy's mom was wearing rolled right down to her ankles. She tried awkwardly to pull them up but only managed to slam her purse into Stacy as they fell to her ankles again. Stacy glanced down at her mother's feet and let out the kind of gasp that grabs everyone's attention. The house lights hadn't gone off quite soon enough.

Before they could agree on what to do or which way to turn, they bounced off each other several times and then "casually" ducked into a row with empty end seats. Stacy's mom kicked off her shoes, pulled the useless limp socks off, and jammed them into her purse. Stacy realized her mom had only replaced one of her shoes on her now bare feet. The other had rolled down the sloping floor to the row of seats in front of them. They bonged heads twice trying to get a look at where it had positioned itself. There was no way they could reach it. The theater was dark and the curtains were about to open. "Ask him, Mom!" she said in reference to the gentleman in front of them. Sheepishly, her mother tapped the elderly man on the shoulder and asked apologetically for her shoe back. Stacy showed me the way her mom's face scrunched up in embarrassment when she asked.

Without another word, they joined a procession of other latecomers as if nothing had happened. But of course something had, and they couldn't forget it.

Flustered and confused, they began climbing the stairs to the balcony section, determined to get away from those in the audience who had witnessed the scene they'd made. But as Stacy followed her mother, she noticed one of the stockings making its way out of the corner of her mom's purse. Mortified that it would be exposed to the audience, or worse yet, land on someone, she took immediate action and wrestled it back inside. "Down boy!" her mother said when she realized what Stacy was doing, and that's when they should have politely removed themselves, but didn't. Stacy and her mother could not stop laughing.

It was difficult maintaining composure as they struggled to their seats. Much to their relief the orchestra hit a crescendo and the appreciative audience clapped loud enough to interrupt the silence and disguise their giggles.

The image of her mom's baggy ankles kept flashing through Stacy's mind, and she lost the battle for composure. The laughter she struggled so desperately to keep down inside erupted like a broken water hydrant. The two of them tried to think about other things, but when one would finally present a calm and poised demeanor, the other would fall apart. The humor of it all seemed impossible to ignore and their emotions too powerful to contain. They laughed so hard it hurt. Stacy said they looked like they were in pain from all the tears of laughter rolling down their cheeks.

More than once Stacy and her mom were mortified when several perturbed adults around them "shhh'd" them and asked for quiet. They didn't blame them for feeling irritated and were ready to bolt at intermission when a man kindly stepped over to them. He said, "I'm thinking about joining you two over here, seems to me you're having a whole lot more fun than I am!"

Stacy told me, "At least someone understood and was nice about it! I'm not sure how we got through it, but we stayed because we really did want to see the ballet."

For a change, Stacy lost her breath from laughing, not from feeling dizzy. She forgot all about her sweaty palms and upset stomach. "The really amazing thing was, it was the first time we've laughed since I was almost killed. I felt like everything was normal and okay again. My mom just looked so ridiculous, I couldn't help it!" ❧

Every now and then for a laugh, Stacy's mom put her baggy ankles on and performed ballerina jumps around the house. The sound of Stacy's laughter was all the reason she needed.

"Trip to Maria Regina"

    On a crisp and beautiful fall morning, my daughter and I drove to a holiday bazaar being held at a monastery for Carmelite nuns. Every year the nuns sell their crafts as a fund-raising event. The outing was my attempt to find some inner peace for myself and my daughter, who seemed so consumed by worry and fear since the burglary in our home. I wanted to show her a way to find relaxation, the way I thought the nuns did—in peace and solitude. I thought we might even sit in the prayer gardens where they were said to regularly "commune with God." I secretly hoped she would want to go there to ask for the courage and safety she had lost as the result of the crime. Our home had been left in a shambles and her prized possessions were stolen or shattered into pieces.

My daughter made it perfectly clear that the only reason she was going with me was to see nuns like the ones in The Sound of Music *and to buy something new.*

We wandered through the main building, shopped for crafts, bought brownies, saw the chapel, peeked in the confession booths, and still, much to our dismay, there wasn't a nun in sight.

We decided to look for the secret gardens. Perhaps the nuns were there. In our zeal to find them, we strayed a bit off the beaten path and discovered some hidden walkways. We knew we were going places we weren't supposed to go. We went down a steep hill with long blades of slippery grass pressed against its side. Growing more and more determined to see what we came for, we continued down an embankment where I imagined we'd find a simple entrance to the gardens. We found the simple entrance and if it hadn't been for the barbed wire fence separating us from it, we would've used it. My daughter nervously asked if I was going to make her climb over it. Worse yet, she wondered half-jokingly if I had plans to dig a tunnel under it, like a convict trying to escape prison, admonishing, "I think it would be a big mistake, Mom."

I assured my daughter that I wasn't about to have searchlights and hound dogs chasing after us in a nun's convent. She looked relieved and told me we would never get back up the hill. I assured her it'd be easy. And I was partially right. She was up it in no time. But I wasn't behind her.

The grass was slick as ice and my boots couldn't get a grip. My daughter, sensing my struggle, ran back and forth to check on my progress, but she tried to keep her distance because, as she said, "there's no sense in both of us getting caught when the nuns find you trying to sneak into their gardens!"

I began making excellent progress on my hands and knees. I might have made it to the top if I had only grabbed a branch that was firmly rooted to a tree. Instead I grabbed one that pulled right out of the ground. I hurled down the hill and landed at the bottom in a heap. I was now in a most unladylike position. My daughter began screaming wildly that I was flashing my underwear to the entire convent.

My daughter continued to laugh excitedly as she ran away. She had no intention of being caught and left me there to face the authorities on my own. Looking down at me from the top of the hill, she made a point of telling me that if the nuns showed up, she had never seen me before in her life.

It wasn't exactly the day I had in mind. Boot camp might have been an easier trip. "You would've been a brave nun, Mom," my daughter said, "but I'm not sure they'd ever take you. It's the same reason I worry about you coming to my school for parent's day, you know?" "Yeah, I get it." I told her. And then she beamed with the biggest smile I had seen on her face in weeks and said "But this was the most fun I've had in a really long time! Especially the part when your skirt blew up!"

When I looked up and saw my daughter watching me as I tried to scale the mountain I was on, I saw delight back in her face. Even in my worst moments in the mud, it was worth losing all my grace and dignity. Like other parents of traumatized children, I was savoring every moment, watching her joy for life return, unabandoned and carefree. Her humor was back.

We left the convent without seeing a nun or sitting in a prayer garden. We left, and a part of her I hadn't seen for way too long came home again. ❧

"Cone Trauma in the Emergency Lane"

❧ *Nothing seemed to please Tommy anymore. Since fire had ravaged his home and destroyed all of his belongings, he felt oddly detached from everything and didn't want anything new. Apathy had settled in over his personality and caused him to withdraw.*

Whenever he was asked a question, Tommy's response was the same, "I don't care."

One evening, Tommy's dad talked him into going out for an ice cream cone. They were his favorite soft cones (chocolate and vanilla "twisties") from a nearby fast-food restaurant. He begged his dad to request nice big ones, complaining that the last few times they had bought them, he noticed they seemed smaller than usual.

He was right. His dad had noticed, too. Both times they left complaining, saying they must have hired a new manager trying to save on ice cream. But Tommy sensed his father's reluctance to complain to the worker, and the more he sensed it, the louder Tommy begged him to say something about it. His father told him, "Absolutely not, that's ridiculous. End of discussion. I won't do it."

Tommy wouldn't stop. He continued driving his point home right up to the ordering microphone. Then his father did what every parenting book warns you not to do—he gave in. He ordered and then politely added that if they could make them a little bigger like they used to, they'd sure appreciate it. Triumphantly, Tommy shouted "Yes! Way to go, Dad!" His father rationalized that it was good to be sure they got their money's worth. He admitted to me that it had been a long time since he had seen his son so motivated about something. "So what if he was a little overzealous about the cone," he decided, "at least he was finally acting like he cared about something."

The worker smiled at them in a funny way when they pulled up to the take-out window. They understood why when they saw what he was about to unload into their car. They were monstrosities, cones the size of footballs. Quarter pound cones or bigger. So huge and so heavy Tommy had to hold his in both hands. They pulled away in shock. They could hear the restaurant staff howling behind them as they left. His dad could barely control the car while holding his cone. "Dad, what are we suppose to do with these things?"

By now, they'd figured out the worker had overheard their exchange at the speaker and was teaching them a lesson. But they had other things to concentrate on. At that moment, the only safe thing to do was get off the road. Tommy's dad said he was thankful to whoever made the decision to put an "emergency only" lane right where he needed one. Probably wasn't the first time something like this happened, they joked.

There they sat. Leaning out both sides of their car with an unidentifiable mass, dripping down their hands, face, and lap, laughing more than eating.

When the realization hit that a police officer could pull over thinking they needed assistance, the hysteria they felt inspired acting aspirations, and they quickly turned into "cops on the beat." Speaking directly into his cone Tommy's dad began, "One Adam twelve, we have a cone trauma in the emergency lane . . . requesting backup please. Over." Tommy continued, "Two male suspects appear to be two real pigs. They've exceeded their limit on twisties and are getting sick all over themselves! Get me some backup, buddy. Ten-four, Over."

They left most of the twisties on the road in two big puddles, looking like two big emergencies. "Burn rubber, Dad," Tommy said coolly, "let's get outta here." It's impossible to "peel out" in a four-cylinder car, but his dad gave it his best shot. As for future twisties, they told me they never asked for anything but a "small" again.

As Tommy and his dad reenacted the story for me they were animated and alive. Humor had managed again to spark a flame in a previously cold and sad heart. This time it would prove to be a flame of restoration, rather than destruction. Humor had moved Tommy a little further along on the road to his healing.

Trauma is never forgotten, and humorous memories can last a life time, too. A sense of humor helps you survive painful times.

Kids Just Want to Have Fun

Children want to have fun as much as they need to have fun. It doesn't change because a traumatic event has taken place. There are times when children will be ready to forget about their pain for a while. When that day comes, be ready. It's good to let yourself "be a kid" again. Join them and let your guard down, too. Sometimes it is good to escape from the hard things in life.

Don't forget to let kids "waste time" now and then. When they're feeling weary, it can help to give them a break from routines and responsibilities. Doing nothing can be fun too.

Have Fun Together

Fun time with your child is important and healing. Play together whenever you can. If you never had time to play before, take time to do it together now. Here are some ideas and some reminders of ways you can have fun together:

- Watch comedies (movies or plays).
- Read light-hearted books.
- Play lively games, requiring some animation.
- Dance around the house, turning up the music.
- Lip-synch to your favorite songs.
- Perform puppet shows.
- Play TV anchorpeople and write your own news for the day.
- Take a bike ride.
- Have a lemonade stand sale or garage sale.
- Build a fort.
- Play musical instruments or sing together.
- Try on clothes you would never really buy.
- Play dress up (pull out old clothes, jewelry, hats).
- Play with a pet.
- Play hair stylist (let your child design your hair).
- Play sports for fun.
- Take a trip to an amusement park.
- Play mad libs (fill-in-the-blank word games) or read joke and riddle books together.
- Sing in funny voices.
- Do anything you and your child consider fun—the sky's the limit.

Humor is good for families. It's the easiest technique you can use to strengthen bonds between you and your children.

Family rituals that bring you together and provide meaning can be invaluable. Families who participate in special activities together create a powerful healing tool for themselves. Placing value and importance on the event they endured and sharing *time together* helps every family member feel valued, important, and needed. Every person plays a role in the recovery of each member of the family.

While the adults set the stage for this form of loving support, family members can all participate in sharing these activities:

- Start a family journal. Keep it in a central location where all can share anything they choose on a daily basis.

- Plan a celebration in which you all acknowledge and celebrate the fact that you survived what you did.

- Plan ceremonies to remember important aspects of your loss. Plant a special tree or flower together in memory. Hold a candle lighting circle to share prayers, memories, or resolutions.

- Write a list of everything you're thankful for and share it with each other.

- Plan trips and vacations that will hold special meaning for everyone.

- Garden together. It is life affirming to begin something new and tend to its progress.

- Read together.

- Volunteer together as a family. Homeless shelters, soup kitchens, churches, and nonprofit agencies abound with opportunities.

- Establish a "family night" each week and take turns choosing the game, movie, or activity you will participate in together. Choosing Sunday nights will give kids something to look forward to at the end of a weekend and may help start the week off in a positive way.

- Don't forget to "date." Married or not, your adult relationships need to be continually nurtured and you need time alone together to do that. Take turns planning and setting up a date at least once a month. Dating time can "refuel" parents and caregivers so they can give back to their kids with increased energy, enthusiasm, and attention.

- Pursue any idea your family creates together.

Remember that recovering from trauma is a continuum. Use humor and laughter to balance the pain. It really works.

7

Healing Through Parenting

"It's too cold, Mommy. I don't want to get wet."

I watched a mother with her daughter down at the edge of a lake one summer evening. The sun was setting and the water was unusually cold. Campfires were springing up all around us to take the chill off the damp air.

The young girl was about six years old and wore shorts and a long-sleeved shirt. She was struggling to put her bare feet in the water and jumped away every time the cold ripples on the water's edge chased her toes. Her mother set down the cup she was holding and suddenly pounced into the water with a huge splash. She howled wildly and then fully submerged herself. She shot up like a rocket and yelled to her daughter, "Come on! It's not cold! You'll get used to it." The little girl replied, "It's too cold, Mommy. I don't want to get wet."

The mother came toward the girl trying to convince her, still yelling, "Come in! You're not cold!" The girl kept insisting she was cold and continued to tell her mother that she did not want to get wet.

Despite my distance I could see her knees knocking as she

hugged herself and began to back away. "Yes, you do!" her mother told her, splashing her with great gusto. The girl screamed and before she could run, her mother grabbed her wrist and doused her again with water. "Please, Mommy, don't! Please don't make me get wet! It's too cold!" she cried. And again her mother replied, "You aren't cold! It feels good, see?"

The helplessness of her tears echoed across the lake. She continued to try to make her mom understand her feelings. She said repeatedly, "I don't like it! Please stop, Mommy, please don't!" Now sobbing, the little girl stood frozen and shivering. Her mom let go of her wrist, but she stood defeated and did not move. Her mother laughed as she continued to ignore her daughter's feelings and splash her with water.

My own daughter caught me fixated on the scene and made the observation that I was spying on people again. She sat down next to me and asked me what had happened. She became as quickly engrossed as I was and together we felt helplessly sad for the young girl. My daughter said to me, "If we can see how she feels all the way across this lake, how come her mom can't?"   ✄

A New and Different Challenge

Some adults are under the mistaken belief that children have it easy. But for many, like the young girl in the example above, childhood is a time of feeling powerless, misunderstood, and shamed. Without the experience of respect and empathy, children are cheated out of resources to help them build resiliency to life's hardships. Even children who haven't been traumatized will have a particularly difficult time learning how to master their young lives without these important parental qualities. When children have the added burden of a trauma to contend with, their resources are even further depleted.

Good parenting goes a long way on the path to children's recovery from trauma. Under an umbrella of respect and empathy, parenting can be healing.

Your ability to parent can change drastically when a trauma has entered your child's life and the life of your family. This chapter is intended to help you gain access to some of the general approaches to parenting you may have lost sight of because of everything you're going through. It may help remind you of ideas and skills you've temporarily lost touch with but can utilize again. Ultimately, these parenting guidelines can be important to the healing of your child after a trauma.

Even under the best of circumstances, parenting is hard work. It brings out the best and the worst in people. At its best, you may feel unconditional love and pure joy just at the sight of your child; at its worst, you may lose your temper, feel frustrated, and worry that you're an awful parent.

Trauma can also bring out the best and worst in your family because of the level of stress, grief, and disruption it has caused all of you. Your parenting style is likely to be challenged in new and different ways, as may the relationships you share with everyone in your family.

Attitudes That Promote Healing

Parenting styles are a critical factor in how children come to terms with what they've been through or resolve what they've heard about or seen. Positive parental attitudes can contribute to children's healing after they've experienced the world in a violent or tumultuous state.

A parental attitude of unconditional acceptance can contribute to your child's healing. When children know your love and acceptance can be depended on, your relationship can act as a safe haven for them in times of trauma. Unconditional acceptance says, "I love you, even when you make mistakes," "I may not accept your behavior, but I will always accept *you*," and "I will always be here for you."

A couple I know have decided they are committed to loving "all of who they are and all of who they aren't." When one of them shows a side that's not particularly easy to be around the other calls out, "All you are, and all you aren't!" It's a reminder to both of them that they have agreed to accept each other's best and worst sides unconditionally. You might try doing this with your family when stress is high. Explain the meaning and purpose of the statement and practice calling it out to each other.

Parenting is an art and a science. If you approach parenting with this attitude, you may be more successful. If you employ artistic qualities like creativity, spontaneity, humor, insight, and compassion, and use scientific skills like rational consequences, consistent methods, and predictable behaviors, your parenting style is more likely to be balanced and effective. Parents who are flexible, creative, and supportive seem to increase their children's resiliency to stress and help their recovery from trauma.

Parenting is hard work. It requires continuous compassion. It can be a thankless and tiring job one day and the most satisfying thing you've ever done the next. Relationships between children and parents are often filled with many highs and lows. They seldom flow smoothly through every stage of development. As children move further away from you and closer to their sense of independence, there are bound to be increased feelings of tension and conflict. It's as normal as babies taking their first step.

Parents who approach parenting with acceptance for the exhaustion it sometimes brings have an easier time when it happens. If the exhaustion you experience prevents you from having the necessary energy to parent at all or causes you to parent with abusive attitudes and behaviors, you owe it to your child and to yourself to seek help immediately.

Does Your Parenting Style Promote or Prevent Healing?

The following questions will help you determine whether or not the qualities you bring to your parenting are a help or a hindrance. If you recognize any of these in yourself, congratulate yourself for achieving an awareness that is necessary to your becoming a healthier, happier parent.

Are you a perfectionist?

Do your children have trouble succeeding in your eyes? If so, you may be passing on to them your unrealistic expectations for their abilities and choices. Parenting and perfection don't mix. If you are disapproving and anxious about everything your children think, say, or do, they may be developing strong feelings of inadequacy. It's important for children to know they can make mistakes and still feel good about themselves. Help children understand that mistakes provide opportunities for growth and learning, not just failure.

Are you able to put yourself in your children's shoes and feel what they may be experiencing?

Do you listen to your child with an ear of empathy? Can you genuinely understand your child's struggles with an empathetic heart? If not, you may lack the ability to nurture the emotional development of your child in the ways he or she needs in order to develop feelings of security and a sense of being loved. A lack of empathy, similar to the one displayed by the mother discussed at the beginning of this chapter who splashed her young daughter with icy cold water, prevents parents from meeting the basic needs of their children.

When feelings and emotions are not honored or acknowledged, a child's development and ability to recover from trauma will be impacted. In such an atmosphere, traumatized children stand little chance of having the safe and predictable environment they need to heal. Instead, they may learn to:

- stop having feelings

- doubt their true feelings

- bury their feelings

- take on other people's feelings

- make life choices based on other people's feelings rather than their own

- feel bad about themselves if their feelings don't match those of others

- isolate themselves because no one seems to understand or believe their feelings

- trust others instead of themselves

In order to heal, traumatized children need empathy. They need to know you can genuinely understand their experience.

Is discipline based on fairness and the result of clearly stated expectations?

Children need to know what to expect from you and what you expect from them. Does punishment reach physical force? Are you fighting for power and control? If physical aggression is your means of gaining your child's attention and obedience, you risk passing down a myriad of confusing and harmful messages and memories to your child.

In the midst of all the stress trauma can create, you may feel like your anger gets the best of you sometimes. Your patience may be stretched to the limit and your own emotions may feel like time bombs ready to explode. It is difficult, if not impossible, to appropriately discipline children when anger is all you have to draw from or use.

If anger is driving your style of discipline, you need professional support to help you learn how to put anger in the back seat and find new emotions and behaviors to carry with you in the driver's seat.

Children's cooperation increases when they are guided by love, given clear directions and expectations, provided firm limits, and redirected with fair and meaningful consequences. You may not be familiar with how to do this if you were not raised this way. There are parenting classes in almost every community that can assist you. All parents need the support of other parents to do a good job and everyone needs access to knowledge and information to be successful.

Do your children parent you?

There's a difference between caring for one another and taking on roles that aren't fair or appropriate. For example, at times when you are ill and your children give helpful caretaking, they have learned how to step in when needed to take responsibility. Perhaps they bring you water or an extra blanket, or maybe they take phone messages to let you sleep. Taking over these responsibilities while you get well shows care and concern for one another. Flexibility is a trait in emotionally thriving families.

However, in families where every problem becomes a crisis, children, as well as their parents, often lose sight of who's in control and who's responsible for what. Pandemonium ensues and often children find themselves taking on adult roles they are not prepared or equipped for.

Some parents find it hard to be adults when life gets hard. There may be many reasons why. Perhaps it is difficult because they also have unmet needs that are critical to their well-being. But children should never be the ones to meet a parent's needs. If this is a problem for you, it is important to learn other ways to take care of yourself. To thrust children into a parent role is to rob them of their childhood. All kids need to live in homes where adults can be the grown-ups. In nurturing families, parents take care of themselves so they can care for their children.

Does your family adhere to a rule of silence?

This can be especially problematic for children trying to come to terms with exposure to trauma. If families as a rule keep each other at an emotional distance, children will learn to hide their pain and guard their feelings. Vital, precious aspects of your child's personality risk being buried. Feelings need to be freely expressed. In nurturing families, feelings can be trusted, understood, expressed, and used in meaningful ways.

Does your child need to make you "look good"?

Sometimes parents make the mistake of seeing children as an extension of themselves, to the point where children are not valued for who they are but for how well they make their parents look. Children who need to make their parents "look good" lose themselves in the process.

Children are unique individuals totally separate from you. Those living in nurturing homes are individually celebrated, honored for unique accomplishments, and treasured for their individuality.

Following trauma, children's feelings, reactions, and needs will not always correspond with yours. Children normally fluctuate in their desire for parental involvement throughout the healing process. Some days they will want to share and be close to you. Other days they will want space and distance. Learn to let your children heal in the ways that work for them, together or apart from you. When independence and self-sufficiency can be exercised, they grow strong and confident.

Nurturing Homes Promote Healing

The special attention you can give children is needed now more than ever. It's important to their comfort and security to have a physical presence through the hard times. Let children know you are there for them. Share your strength through the difficult times.

In the second grade I sat next to Millie, a girl who repeatedly witnessed violence in her home. I knew it, the adults around her knew it, but nothing was ever done about it. When she threw up all over our desk at the same time every day, her background was the least of my worries. After lunch, I had learned to move all papers and books off the top of our desk and put supplies on the shelf below. Then I would brace myself for what was to come. And when it came, I helped with the clean-up and did my best to protect my belongings. Some days I went for the janitor, other days I walked with her to the nurse's office. Most of the time I went for paper towels and a paper cup filled with water for her to sip. Not long after that, I developed a lifelong aversion to people's upset stomachs and avoided them like the plague. And then I became a parent.

Some of the times my child has needed me the most have been when she was about to throw up, when she was throwing up, and after, when she was getting ready to throw up again. My physical presence was what she needed most. I became highly skilled at holding hair, washcloths, and bags at the same time. I devised ingenious distractions for myself when the retching continued beyond even what motherly love could bear. But I did it all because it helped an otherwise helpless situation. And besides, it was a small price to pay compared to what she was going through.

I often think back to Millie, the little blond waif of a girl who sat next to me and suffered every day without the physical presence of her mother or father. Looking back, I'm sure I was selected as her deskmate because I didn't scream and add to her embarrassment like others in the class. I was tolerant, but silently I hated it just as much as anyone else. I accepted it though, because I somehow knew it was out of her control and I liked her.

I remember how Millie dropped her head so strands of hair hid her face. I knew she felt ashamed, and I tried to keep talking to her as if it were no big deal, but she needed more than the advice I had to offer. She needed to hear that she deserved to be safe at home and that it was okay to call the police or another adult to help her when it wasn't. She needed to hear that someone was going to protect her. She needed to hear that she was not bad, it was not her fault, and she had good reasons for losing her lunch. She needed to be told that what was happening around her and to her was wrong. Instead she got my advice, an eight-year-old's words of wisdom: "Try chewing your food up better next time. Maybe it won't happen again if you chew more." It was the only advice I knew to give. Years later the family violence in Millie's home finally came out into the open. But it came too late for her siblings, who suffered a violent death at the hands of Millie's mother.

I'm grateful I tried to show Millie some compassion through my actions, but I knew even then that nothing could replace the presence of a loving parent. And I knew she didn't have that presence, not at school or anywhere around her.

Nurturing homes are abuse-free homes. Love makes it easy to nurture your children even when it's hard. After trauma, even though children may not be physically ill, they need you by their side to nurse them back to health. They need your loving presence.

Parents Don't Have to Be Perfect

You don't have to be a perfect parent to have a happy family or to love your child with all your heart. You don't have to be a perfect parent before a trauma or after a trauma in order for your child to heal.

As human beings we are naturally going to be imperfect. This is a fact of life. The only difference between a family that's working well together and one that's not are the attitudes and expectations of the parents guiding it. Parents in happy families cope with their mistakes. They are open about their faults and admit when they are wrong. They face their imperfections and model healthy self-acceptance for their children. They teach their children how to learn from mistakes and find honor in being accountable for them.

Parents in nurturing homes role model change, acceptance, flexibility, forgiveness, love, and acceptance of their own shortcomings. Happy families also know how to stay connected to each other, even after a trauma. I have one question I ask to see if a family is connected or not. Do you have fun together? If you can't remember the last time you really laughed, relaxed, and played with your child, it's the next thing you need to do. Don't wait. Go have fun. If you don't know how, just ask your child what they'd like to do.

Love can keep growing and developing if you stay connected to each other and stay open about your imperfections. These characteristics in parents help kids heal. Coming to terms with tragedy requires you to simply be honest, open, and human with your kids. It's so much easier than striving for perfection.

When Anger Hits Home: Power Struggles, Revenge Fantasies, and Aggression

When a child's inner conflicts are wrapped in anger, behaviors may be expressed that disrupt family relationships and harmony. Power struggles, revenge fantasies, and aggression are behaviors you may need to contend with. For some parents, it is extremely challenging to cope with these effects of trauma. For others, it is a parenting nightmare. The more you understand, the better chance you have of knowing what to do. Although helpful to many, prevention techniques and deescalating strategies are not always enough. Get professional help for children if anger is dangerous or persistently present.

Power Struggles

After a trauma, it is not uncommon for children to feel they have to fight and argue with you or others in order to regain a sense of power and control. They may refuse to comply with your decisions, disobey your rules, and become defiant over seemingly minor requests. You may find yourself instantly embroiled in a heated debate that only escalates with every reason and justification you give. It's not uncommon to lose sight of the original disagreement when a slew of complaints are added to a boiling kettle of conflict. Suddenly, everyone is on trial for something and must prove themselves right or risk an unfair "guilty" verdict.

Power struggles often escalate into damaging forms of communication:

- They put down others rather than build others up.

- They blame and shame rather than acknowledge mistakes and express acceptance.

- They express sarcasm rather than real feelings.

- They criticize rather than hold realistic expectations.

- They lash out with anger rather than express what is hurtful.

It is normal for kids to need to regain a sense of personal empowerment after trauma, but clearly power struggles won't help them find it. If children are challenging you by engaging in them, the best antidote is to support their need for power and provide opportunities for them to get it back. Make it possible for them to experience more power and control so they won't have to fight for it.

Resist the impulse to become more controlling in the midst of a power struggle. Instead, negotiate and be firm with your limits and expectations. For instance, you can respond to a child refusing to do his homework by saying something like this:

- I can understand why you'd rather be doing something else right now. What are you going to do when you're finished with your homework?

- You don't have to like doing it, but you need to finish your homework anyway.

- It sounds like a lot of hard work. What do you think is the best way to start?

- I wish you didn't have homework, either! I was hoping we could do something fun, maybe you could finish it so we could still have time to play!

- I know you are good at doing what you need to do, even when you don't feel like it. It's hard to get started sometimes. What would help you to start?

- Some days are really tough. You have a lot to do and it must feel overwhelming. Why not take a break and come back to it when you're ready?

You will do better if you can be creative with your child's challenging behavior while utilizing sound skills. It's up to you to step back and refuse to engage in a struggle.

Listening Skills Can Help

Better communication starts with using your ears, not your mouth. Good listening increases the chances that you will experience a fair discussion rather than step into a battle to "win" a power struggle with your child. Skillful listening will help you diffuse escalating arguments and draw people together instead of apart.

When Jake witnessed a robbery at a local convenience store, his fear continued to interfere with his life for months afterwards. His parents didn't believe that Jake could still be struggling with so much fear. They concluded that he was saying he still felt afraid because he wanted to get out of going to bed. This is what followed:

Jake: I don't want to go to bed. That show made me scared.

Parent: It wasn't scary. You shouldn't be scared by that. Quit stalling and get to bed.

Jake: But I can't! You need to come with me!

Parent: Stop acting like a baby. You're old enough to go to bed by yourself!

Jake: But I'm scared!

Parent: Well don't be! There's nothing to be scared of! Don't make excuses!

Jake: I'm not! You can't make me go to bed!

Parent: Get to bed this instant, or no more television for a week.

Jake: I hate you!

Parent: Now you're grounded!

When adults don't know how to tune in differently to their children, their reactions can escalate conflict. In the next scenario, Jake's parents learned how to put listening skills into action. The outcome was cooperation and the opportunity for Jake to feel a sense of respect.

Jake: I don't want to go to bed. That show made me scared.

Parent: Scary shows do that sometimes. They might make it hard for you to want to go to sleep. What do you feel worried or scared about?

Jake: I don't know.

Parent: Scary feelings are hard to understand sometimes. Since it's time for you to get into bed now, I wonder what you could do to help yourself feel less afraid?

Jake: You could read me a story.

Parent: What a good idea. Reading a happy story can help you feel less afraid. I can read to you for ten minutes. After that, you can read to yourself for another five minutes if you still want to. That's a very smart way to handle your scary feelings.

This scenario could have gone many different ways, but the initial response to Jake conveyed an attitude of respect, concern, and belief. Conflict was diffused and Jake's parents helped him learn how to problem solve.

You might be wondering, "But what if Jake really was stalling and wasn't really scared? Should you let him manipulate his parents in this way?" Regardless of whether or not Jake was really feeling scared or not, he was listened to and was encouraged to find ways to come up with solutions to a problem. The discussion did not end up in a power struggle, but rather led to positive problem solving. It was also an opportunity for Jake to find a way to cope with future feelings of fear. In the long run, these benefits far outweigh the drawbacks to allowing him to stay up an extra fifteen minutes.

Assume your child is telling the truth. It may be important to check out feelings if you have a hunch there is more going on or they are having difficulty being truthful with you. But remember, all children try out different methods for trying to get what they want or need. It's normal. Accept that your child will exaggerate the truth sometimes and help them find a way to express what really is going on inside them. Help them learn how to tell the truth, so it will be easier next time.

If Jake's parents wanted to address whether or not he was actually feeling afraid or was really wanting something else, they could encourage an honest response by saying something like this:

> I wonder if what you are really wanting is more time with me. Telling me you're scared or sick or sad might seem more important, but wanting to have more time with me just because you want to is important, too. I want to be with you, too. Let's figure out a way we can spend more time together before bedtime. Maybe you could get ready for bed earlier so we could read an extra book or play a game.

Always keep your statements tentative when exploring questions you have about your child's feelings. Remember, your child knows better than anyone what he or she is feeling. Help your child believe this, too.

Encourage children to discover their own answers to a problem by getting them involved in finding their own solutions. Give them the message, "You are capable." A proactive attitude helps kids get their sense of personal power back without having to fight you for it. A proactive parenting approach is a powerful tool for healing.

Revenge Fantasies

It is important to distinguish between fantasies and reality. "Fantasies" of revenge are not actually plans for revenge. If children have the intent or a plan for revenge, immediate professional intervention is required. The revenge fantasies discussed here exist in a child's make-believe world, expressed through play or art.

Children can be afraid of their own anger. When they have an opportunity to play out fantasies of revenge, children can reenact their fears and work through memories of the tragedy in a safe way. When children are not a risk to themselves or others, it is important to tolerate playful acts of revenge and not punish or try to tone down feelings of rage.

Revenge fantasies take many different forms. Children may write letters to those they wish revenge on, dream about ways to find revenge, or act out an array of possibilities to make those responsible "pay." Adults are often alarmed when they witness children playing out fantasies of revenge, but children who do are generally moving closer to healing.

Cody drew me two pictures of the drunk driver who killed his mom. In the first drawing the offender was hit and run over by a car. He told me he wanted what happened to his mom to happen to the man who killed her. In the second drawing, he placed the offender inside a locked jail cell, stabbed and bleeding profusely from the heart. Cody drew himself standing nearby and laughing as he hung the keys to the cell over a toilet he was about to flush.

Cody's anger needed expression, and his revenge fantasies helped him experience some control over the powerlessness he felt when the offender in this case was let out of jail. Cody's feelings of revenge didn't last long, but they helped him accept his feelings about a difficult situation in the only way he knew how.

Aggression

Anger and aggression are not the same thing. Anger is a feeling and aggression is a behavior. Explain the difference to your child and help him or her transform the weapon of anger into a tool for positive growth and healthy expression. To do this you will need to know when to intervene and help your child learn to express anger constructively.

Often children are looking for adults around them to set limits and help them stay safe. When impulse control is a problem they may be asking for you to take more control for them. This must always be done in ways that do not physically hurt or intimidate them. In time, discipline that is based on fairness, predictability, and love will teach your child the value of respect and the joy of making healthy choices.

Parents often ask why a trauma causes some children to become aggressive. Every child's experience is different, but here are some possible explanations for why children choose aggression:

- It's an attempt to strike out at what happened.

- It's an attempt to punish the one(s) who caused the hurt.

- It's a way to express and cope with feelings of helplessness and fear.

- It's an attempt to understand what happened.

- It's a way to reenact what was done to them.

- It's a way to distract themselves from painful feelings.

- It's an attempt to regain power and control.

- It's a way to forget whatever else is troubling them.

- It's a way to look and feel powerful so they might be less vulnerable to it happening again.

Even though your child may be expressing anger in ways you've never seen from them before, it's important not to try to stifle their angry feelings. Aggressive behaviors need your intervention, but feelings need to be expressed.

You and your friends and relatives may tire of hearing your child express intense feelings of anger, but expressing them is an alternative to acting on them. As a parent, your goal is to help your children express anger to the person they need to, by telling them directly how they feel, for the right purpose, and in the right way, free of physical and verbal attacks.

Here are some suggestions of things you can do and say to children when they're experiencing anger and aggression:

- "It's not okay to hit when you feel angry. You need to take a time-out. When it's over you can apologize and tell me with words why you're mad."
- "You can feel mad without hurting yourself or anyone else."
- "It's okay to feel mad and think what to do."
- "It's okay to feel angry, but you have to control how you act."
- Encourage your child to say what is upsetting them. Ask, "What do you feel angry about? What is it you are most furious about?"
- Ask them to draw a picture of what their anger looks like or what makes them feel angry. (Then ask them to describe and explain their drawings.)
- Ask, "If your fist could talk instead of hit, what would it say?"
- Disengage and stay calm. Discover what is behind your child's anger. Ask yourself what your child might feel hurt about, or if he or she is really afraid, lonely, exhausted, or hungry?
- Respond rather than react. Productive anger takes the form of a dialogue. Help your children give voice to anger and *respond* to their needs the best you can.

Try to help your children replace a negative behavior with a positive one. Show your kids a variety of healthy ways to express anger without aggression. Give children ideas for new coping behaviors. You might say, "It's okay to feel angry. Here's what to do with it . . ." Here are some suggestions:

- Help them talk their feelings through.
- Turn them to directed physical activity to reduce tension (i.e. hitting tennis balls, weeding, walking the dog, jogging, cleaning, sports).
- Suggest that they take time alone.
- Suggest that they stay with their anger for a while and notice how it feels.

- Sign your children up to participate in martial art classes that teach self-discipline, control, respect, and self-confidence.

- Encourage journal or diary writing.

- Suggest that they try writing poetry or uncensored letters to whoever or whatever they want.

- Encourage them to express their feelings through art.

- Tell them it's healthy to cry.

- Suggest that they count to ten or one hundred when they feel angry.

- Let them rip up an old phone book.

Explain to your children that as long as they don't hurt themselves or anyone else, they can do what helps them the most. It is important to help kids understand that letting go of anger does not mean they have to forget what happened or pretend everything's okay.

Sometimes you can help children resolve feelings of anger through humor and laughter. This only works when no one is teased, ridiculed, or embarrassed in the process. Make sure you can laugh at yourself first, and then laugh *with* your children, not *at* them.

Unsafe Behaviors

Help children understand that it is never okay when their behavior is hurtful, dangerous, or unsafe to themselves or others. If children's actions or play turns to direct violence against another, an animal or themselves, it must be immediately stopped and talked about. Immediate, consistent, and firm intervention is needed. Seek professional intervention to learn how to help your child contain unsafe behaviors and learn why they're happening.

You will never be able to prevent all of your child's misbehavior, but you can redirect it in helpful ways when it happens. Role model self-acceptance for your own mistakes to help your children own up to theirs. Do not shame children for losing control, but instead guide them and encourage them to respond differently next time. Express confidence in their ability to change aggressive behavior and learn from their mistakes.

Common Challenges for Parents

If a trauma has hurt your child physically, emotionally, and spiritually, it has hurt you, too. It can be challenging to cope with your own reactions to what has happened to them. Seek professional support if you need help with feelings of rage and retaliation, guilt and self-blame, fear for your child that leads to overprotectiveness, marital and relationship strain, or an inability to attend to your other children.

Children need to be able to count on you to maintain self-control and to show them how to cope with anger without retaliation or other dangerous behaviors. You need to move past feelings of guilt and self-blame so these emotions won't divert you from your children's needs. Children need your help to regain self-confidence and independence. If you are overprotective of them, they may worry more and be discouraged from participating in activities that could help them overcome their fears. Don't deny your children's independence even after a trauma.

Tremendous strain on relationships can also occur after a trauma. When tension and arguing are consistently present in your marriage or adult relationships, feelings of insecurity may increase in your child. Blaming each other causes a child to believe he or she is to blame, too.

Another thing to be aware of is that it is easy to spend all your energy on the child most greatly impacted by the traumatic event and ignore the needs of other children in your family. Every child in your home has been greatly impacted and needs special support at this time. Let all children know their needs are just as important to you. Plan special time with each one.

Some Days It's Hard to Be a Family

Pain is more bearable when it is shared. Families can be a source of strength to one another in the aftermath of trauma. Your family can be one of the most powerful sources of support you'll ever find. Children need supportive relationships in order to heal from trauma, but what if your family has always experienced more chaos than support? If your family relationships were problematic before the trauma ever happened, you may wonder how you will ever get through this now.

Family Chaos

There are days in the life of every family that are filled with disorder and conflict. But when trauma increases the chaos in a family that already lives in a chronic state of disorder, it can lead to serious problems in relationships between parents and children.

"Dysfunctional family" is a popular term used today to describe families that are hurtful to one another in a variety of ways. One of the preoccupations family members have in dysfunctional homes is to tear each other down rather than build each other up.

It may be blatant or subtle, but in a dysfunctional family you will hear people blaming and shaming each other in persistent ways. Children growing up in these families may believe they are somehow defective and unlovable. They often don't feel loved for who they are and feel shamed for who they aren't. Without help, a traumatized child living in such a family may be prevented from ever healing. The effects last long into adulthood, and like a chain reaction, these children will often hurt others in their path.

Family members are bound to see life from different points of view. Mood swings and personality variations make family life a challenge for everyone. If the tension in your home is high enough and lasts long enough, you and your children need to consider ways to change an environment that is painful and depressing to everyone.

When hurt feelings are dealt with openly it is an opportunity to grow closer. Being honest and explaining yourself truthfully can go a long way to building bridges between you. If you find it difficult to talk to one another, try writing your feelings to each other for a while. It takes time and practice to learn different ways of communicating.

Seeing life from different points of view is one thing. If someone in the family has a serious problem with an addiction of any kind, mood swings or personality changes that are difficult or frightening to live with, financial and job stress, or anger that is intimidating or unsafe to others or pets, it needs to be faced before communication skills can significantly help you. Confront the real problem in yourself or your partner. Talk to someone who is able to stay objective and help you think of a solution. Friends can come up with advice they think you should follow, but professional support and intervention is usually needed when you are facing serious issues impacting everyone in your family. Don't delay getting help. Your family is worth whatever it will take to heal.

When You Feel Estranged from Your Children

It is painful to feel emotionally and physically alienated from your children. You may be so tired of conflict that you find that there are days when you dislike your children. You might feel guilty and ashamed about the way you feel about them. Keep in mind that your children probably feel the same way about you. No one feels satisfied when everyone is frustrated.

What to Do When You Need Help

You may be at a point where you feel your family itself is defective. Perhaps you are angry and resentful that yours is not the family you had always dreamed of having. You may envy other families because they seem happier than yours. You may feel you have failed as a parent. Plenty of families experience difficulties like these, and the ones who resolve their problems are the ones who seek help.

Parent Education and Counseling

You may need help to learn how to become a more nurturing parent and family. If you do, you are not alone. All parents can at one time or another benefit from someone else's experience, training, or approach. Be open to others helping you. Even if you're a single parent, you don't have to do it all single-handedly.

There are cultural influences and physiological and hereditary factors intertwined in many behavior problems and challenges that families must face. But if you are committed to being the best parent you can be, there is a lot you can do to change and improve your parenting skills.

It's important to examine what needs changing in yourself before you can make changes in your family. Sometimes it is your own discomfort with certain feelings that cause you to react to your kids in nonhelpful ways.

Parent education and counseling can teach you ways to parent differently than the way you might have been parented yourself. Like a marriage or partnership, parent/child relationships require attention, time, respect, and commitment. Counseling can offer insights to increase your awareness and understanding of reasons you behave and feel the way you do toward your children. It can help you learn ways to stop reenacting hurtful behaviors you may have been subjected to in the past.

Seeking assistance can help you access your strengths as a parent and learn how to respond to your kids as the unique and special individuals they are. With help, you can watch the relationship you have with your children transform. Bring out the best in yourself so you can bring out the best in your children.

Family Counseling

A professional therapist might recommend counseling for your whole family. Going together can be an opportunity to learn new ways to help each other through difficult times. For some families it will be the first time they have shared feelings or cried together about the trauma that impacted them. You may learn things about your family members that you didn't know before.

Working together in counseling can help change negative family habits by shaking them up a bit. Ways of talking, teasing, or giving put-downs may be challenged and replaced. Family counseling can deepen your bonds. You may discover a new sense of appreciation for "all you are and aren't."

Your Self-Care

It can be difficult for parents and adults to carry on the chores and responsibilities of a household while coping with the effects of trauma on their children.

In addition to seeking support through parent education and professional counseling, it is important to be mindful of all the ways you can practice self-care on a daily basis that require little or no expense. Here are twelve ways to help you balance the demands:

1. *Lower your expectations of yourself.* It's okay not to do it all.

2. *Don't make any major changes or decisions right now.* Give yourself time.

3. *Put off what you can and ask for help with what you can't.* Learn to accept help from others so you can have more time to spend with your children.

4. *Don't isolate yourself from your kids or from people who care.* It can be frightening for children to see you withdrawn or immobilized. They need to be connected to you and a variety of adults who care about them.

5. *Give yourself a break and prepare your children in advance.* It's normal for kids to have strong fear of abandonment following trauma. Explain why you are giving yourself a break, how long it will be for, and who will care for them. Unless there are safety issues, don't send children away or leave for long periods of time.

6. *Stress is fatiguing, so get plenty of rest and maintain normal sleep schedules and a healthy diet.* Moderate exercise can also help

counteract feelings of depression, as can treating yourself to something that helps you feel good about yourself.

7. *Don't self-medicate.* Alcohol and nonprescription drugs can lead to destructive coping behaviors and interfere with your ability to parent. Let a physician carefully assess what, if any, medications might be helpful to you.

8. *Normal routines are not only reassuring to children, they can be stabilizing for you, too.* When day-to-day tasks continue, it can help you stay focused and help you live with a continued sense of purpose.

9. *Share your strength.* Show your kids how to regain control of life by helping them with tasks and by giving support and playtime with them. Remember to balance what you do for others with the time and energy you give to yourself.

10. *Make sure you spend enough alone time with your partner or friends who care about you.* Maintain and protect relationships that are separate from your kids. Make time for your own social and/or spiritual life. A break from the parental role will be needed and can be refreshing.

11. *Use paper and pen. Writing can be a healthy outlet for all the emotions, fears, and challenges you face.* It's a positive way to let go of and put away disturbing, confusing and powerful thoughts and feelings.

12. *Give to yourself.* Give yourself a treat, such as flowers, quiet time, magazines, books, movies, walks, music, massages, pedicures, or a therapy session.

Your children are depending on you for stability and strength, but overextending yourself to help others—even your children—will not help anyone. Taking care of your own emotional well-being will help them find theirs. It's part of the balancing act of parenting.

Some Final Guidelines

After a life-changing event, keep the following guidelines in mind:

- *Stay involved with your child.* However you do this is fine, just keep doing it. Share bedtime stories, attend band concerts and soccer games, watch a movie together, take a bike ride, or help with homework.

- *Prepare children for how the trauma will affect them personally.* In addition to the emotional effects, explain any time or financial difficulties that you anticipate.

- *Be consistent with what you say and what you do.* Let your kids know they can depend on you. Reassure them that you will be truthful with them. Let them know they can trust you. Answer questions simply and directly. Make sure they understand what you are saying. Follow through with the commitments you make and avoid making promises you can't keep.

- *Know your priority.* Make your children your priority. Children develop self-worth and respect for themselves when they are given positive time and attention from you. Opportunities to listen to all that's on their mind happen every day—actively seek them out and make them happen.

- *Direct and guide.* After a crisis it may be important to relax some rules in your home. Keep your expectations reasonable, but at the same time tell children what you want them to remain responsible for. Let them know what you continue to expect from them in terms of chores, homework, and behavior. Continual structure provides kids safety and security.

- *Maintain normal discipline.* Children need you to be in control now more than ever. Everyone in the family needs to adhere to the structure and rules of the home despite what happened. Don't be afraid to set limits around inappropriate behavior and remember to separate the behavior from your child. For example you might say, "I want to be with you, but I don't like the way you are hitting right now." Maintain discipline by using meaningful consequences that help children learn to change inappropriate behaviors. For example your consequence(s) for hitting might be: You stop playing with them; they have a time-out until they can change their behavior; they might join you again when they can apologize and use their words instead of their fists; you acknowledge and set up a reward each time they use their words instead of their fists; and/or they may return to play when they can identify a different action to take besides hitting.

- *Educate the people your child has regular contact with.* In addition to your child's teacher, you may need to help day care workers, baby-sitters, coaches, and others understand how your child has been affected by the trauma. Work closely with those who may be able to offer your child added support at this time.

- *Let kids be kids, recovering at their own pace.* Following a trauma, don't tell children they must be brave or strong. Let them be children. In the aftermath of trauma kids not only need to slow down, they should slow down. Don't expect them to maintain their normal pace. It takes time to get your bearings and kids deserve your patience while they are trying to get theirs.

- *Children need playtime.* Plan regular time for your children to play or just hang out with their friends. It is beneficial for kids to participate in their usual activities. Some will choose to resume normal activities right away while others will want to give themselves a little more time. Let your children be your guide in this respect.

Parenting in a Violent World

Everywhere you turn, it seems, violence is being pushed on kids. Violence has become celebrated entertainment. It is challenging for parents to teach children nonviolent ways of being in the world when so many others glorify it and when they are so easily exposed to it in their lives.

We crave easy answers to difficult problems, but none exist. Prevention of violence requires interventions at many different levels. An important step parents can take to prevent violence is to protect children from witnessing it daily. Parents may want to carefully screen or refuse to watch television shows, movies, or music videos, or play games or read materials that glorify violence and hate. You can teach your children about behaviors that are unacceptable in real life and tell them why. The way you live and the choices you make will impact the life choices your children will make.

You can help children understand it is strong and courageous to choose peaceful solutions to conflict, and in the process they will become part of the solution to violence, rather than part of the problem.

In April, 1999, a school was ambushed by gunfire in Littleton, Colorado. Fifteen lives were lost and many more were wounded. Following this catastrophic event, threats of more violence began to ripple through schools in almost every state throughout the nation. Rumors about more violent destruction, death threats, and signs of hate quickly spread, increasing children's fears about attending school and parents, anxiety about sending them. In some cases these rumors and threats began to thrive in a climate of panic and hysteria. The struggle for understanding could be felt everywhere.

In the speaking engagements and training's I provided during this time I was repeatedly asked, "Why are so many of our children suddenly making *more* of these threats? What is becoming of our nation's youth?" The disappointment, sense of loss, and hopelessness filled every room I spoke to. The underlying question seemed to be: What is it about our homes, schools, and culture that is producing such imbedded roots of hate in the hearts and minds of our youth? And more importantly, what can we do about it?

I was lecturing one afternoon about the, tendency of traumatized children to reenact what they've witnessed or been exposed to through their play, art, and behaviors, I explained that when surrounded by atrocities they cannot comprehend, children may choose behaviors that reflect their fears and reenact what they can't make sense of. It occurred to me that one possible explanation or contributing factor in the rash of threats assaulting our schools was due to the intense fear and confusion students everywhere were experiencing. Perhaps, I concluded, our youth were acting out the troubling thoughts and feelings that had no where else to go.

On a national level it seemed as though children's sense of powerlessness and fear was being replaced by acts of verbal and physical aggression in a misguided attempt for self-protection and control. If my theory was even partially correct, it became clear to me that children were in desperate need of a supportive environment in which they could be free to ask difficult questions and acknowledge and express their painful thoughts and feelings. They needed help restoring a sense of stability in their world. Without such an environment, children are often left to their own resources and may align with the very behaviors that frighten them the most.

It bears repeating that adults need to be ready to openly talk, listen, guide, comfort, and support children through times of uncertainty. In addition to supporting the hearing process in general, the guidelines outlined in this book may also help prevent children from choosing cruel and dangerous ways to voice their pain.

Parental intervention is not the only answer, but with your help, children can often learn to manage the overwhelming effects of such atrocities in constructive ways, without causing further verbal or physical harm to themselves and others. It is best to seek professional help for additional support and guidance.

8

Healing Is an Everyday Miracle

"My family has peace again."

Amanda said she use to love everything about the wind. She enjoyed running outside on windy days just to feel the strength of the air against her face and feel her hair take flight, wild and out of control. She liked to hear the wind howling in the middle of the night, blowing the rain against her window pane. She told me she use to think the wind was exciting. But now, she said, it would never feel that way again.

Amanda and her family quickly prepared themselves for the hurricane that was about to descend upon their community. They knew what to do and where to go to protect themselves. The emergency shelter they evacuated to had been previously prepared. But when it was safe to leave, no one was prepared for the devastation they would see and the wreckage they would find. The hurricane had beaten down and destroyed a large portion of their community.

Amanda's family searched in vain for the familiar landscaping and lamppost that once stood outside their home. Amanda kept thinking they were on the wrong street because nothing looked right. They found the house they had filled with years of fond memories plummeted to the ground. Amanda's mom and dad started to cry. Amanda held her younger brother's hand and felt shaky and sad.

Amanda and her family came to counseling a few weeks later. Her father said, "The hurricane tore apart our lives and the kids are having a hard time. We're all having trouble with it."

Since it happened, Amanda's six-year-old brother, Michael, had been unable to sleep through the night. He was experiencing nightmares that woke everyone in a panic. He screamed and cried out repeatedly in the night and was tearful through the day. Michael believed the hurricane was an "angry monster" that ate his favorite toys. In a counseling session with his sister, Michael began to mourn the loss of his teddy bear named "Freddie." As he spoke about the stuffed animal he couldn't find in time to take with him to the emergency shelter, he tightened the grip he had on his soft fleece vest and crawled up into his sister's lap. He told me, "I want us to move to someplace underneath the ground before the angry monster comes back again."

Amanda refused to unpack her belongings in the apartment they were temporarily living in. She preferred to leave everything she had received in boxes because she didn't know how long it would be hers anyway. She told me, "I keep thinking it'll just happen again so I don't really want to get use to my new stuff. Besides, I don't like this place. It feels uncomfortable and I don't think it's built very strong." Amanda listened for signs of weakness in the walls and roof every time the weather seemed to be changing. Sometimes she thought she heard the wind picking up speed in the middle of a calm, still night. She asked, "What if we wouldn't have made it to the shelter in time? If we hadn't, the same thing that happened to our house would've happened to us. I feel like I need to stay awake for the rest of my life so I can be ready when it happens again."

Amanda's mother and father were worried, too. They described being in the grips of one argument after another. Amanda's father said, "I know we should be grateful to have our lives, and I am grateful, but I have to wonder, what kind of life is this?" The financial uncertainty, upheaval, and stress the whole family experienced was like no other situation they had ever faced. Amanda's mother said, "I just want it to be like it used to be. I want all of us to be happy again. A part of me thinks we'll be okay, but another part is afraid we won't."

Everything Amanda's parents had once believed to be secure was now thrown into doubt. Their jobs, finances, home, relationship, and entire future were disrupted with uncertainties. The impact on

Amanda's parents was overwhelming at times. They disagreed on steps to take with their children and argued adamantly about whether to relocate or not and whether to make career changes. The spiritual beliefs they assumed would always hold them together felt weakened now. Amanda's parents worried that their relationship would be another casualty in the storm and feared for the overall security of their family.

Through the course of couple counseling, Amanda's parents frequently expressed a sense of hopelessness and despair for the future and for their marriage. Some days they felt like giving up. Because they didn't, they eventually learned how to adjust to the changes the hurricane had forced into their lives.

As counseling continued, Amanda's parents learned ways to accept the full range of their emotions and the normalcy of their reactions and found ways to help their children do the same. They discovered how to pull together, support, and comfort each other rather than isolate and avoid each other. The family needed to share, support, and find new ways to find joy together again. When they did, the bonds of their love were strengthened. The focus of their thoughts and feelings moved away from the hurricane's destructive forces and progressed toward the appreciation they felt for one another. Their love, they concluded, had grown deeper because they were forced to rely on it. "It's a miracle we got through all this. We finally just decided the hurricane took enough from us. We weren't going to let it take our family too."   ✌

Recovering from a traumatic event feels like a miracle. In the midst of a life-altering experience it hardly feels possible that life will ever be normal again. As impossible as it may seem, recovery does happen. Bearing witness to the healing process in children and their families has been one of my greatest privileges over the past fifteen years.

The Road to Healing

There are many personal and professional roads to healing. You may have traveled through the emotions, thoughts, and fears your child has shared with you. You may have offered comfort and parental first aid along the way. You may have also taken professional roads that led you to counseling and therapeutic treatment for your child, yourself, and your family. Parent education and support may have aided your journey. Children need help finding the road to healing. They aren't likely to recover unless the adults in their lives show them how to reach their destination and how to continue beyond.

Healing can be a long, ongoing journey with many delays, setbacks, and stops along the way. At different stages of development, children may need to go back and travel some of the same roads again. Child expert Lenore Terr also believes new problems may develop related to the trauma as a new phase of development appears (Terr 1989). As the level of their understanding changes and matures, children may want to learn more about what happened. They may grow more curious about details and circumstances that led up to and followed the incident. Children will need your help and encouragement as they seek to identify new thoughts and feelings. They will benefit from your ability to listen to their questions every step of the way. All children need adults to be honest with them through all the stages of their development.

If proper help and support have been made available to your children, you can reassure them that even though the memory may remain in years to come, it will never hurt to the degree it did when it happened.

The Gift of Recovery

It is through the connection children have with others that the healing process begins. Inform your kids, friends, teachers, and relatives about the reactions to trauma that are common and normal. The more support children receive from family members, friends, and those initially responding to them, the sooner their difficulties will diminish.

Buried pain leads to many confusing feelings in adulthood. Continue to teach your children ways to release pain rather than bury it. Your reactions and guidance through this process can leave longlasting impressions. Parents who share their children's grief and offer an empathetic response to all their thoughts and feelings, can help children build resiliency to stress and strengthen their ability to cope with difficult times in the future.

Children perceive and react to trauma in many different ways, but following a life-altering event, many will change their ideas about their life or future. It is difficult to make sense out of a senseless act or situation. Children who have healed come to the understanding that while the world can be unsafe, all of life is not dangerous. However, regaining this trust and hope in the world will not be an easy process. Responding in ways that will help children find meaning in their experiences is rarely easy, but adults who create a safe environment for children to openly question, express, and feel are on the right track.

After nine-year-old Steven witnessed a car accident in his neighborhood, he developed a fear of driving in cars. He told me, "It makes me worried every time my family is in our car. Even when I'm not with them I'm afraid they won't come back! That happens you know. People get killed in their cars and their families never see them again." "Yes that does happen," I said. "It's very sad when it does, and it's hard to make sense of it. Accidents like the one you saw don't usually happen. Most adults are safe drivers. But when accidents do happen, it's wonderful how many people know what to do to help. Grown-ups like police officers, firefighters, and ambulance drivers are trained to know exactly what they need to do, so most people can get better if they've been hurt." We talked about all the precautions that are taken when driving in a car, including the use of seat belts and following the rules of the road.

Steven's parents helped him understand that people can control a lot of what happens in their cars, but that mistakes happen, too. They told him, "We expect to be alive for a long, long time, but if something were to happen to us there would be grown-ups to help you in our place." His parents made a point of explaining more of the safety measures they took as they were driving and assured him they would always do everything in their power to drive safely and protect themselves, their children, and everyone else in the car with them. They continually reassured him by saying, "We love you and will do everything in our power to keep you and ourselves safe."

Children and adults feel and think differently, react uniquely, and cope in a variety of ways; but in the end, trauma can bond you together. Your support and companionship throughout your child's recovery is a testimony to your love.

Recovery is a gift. It may appear when you least expect it. And often it is a pleasant surprise. It brings relief and peace to the heart, to the mind, to the body, and to the soul. It means resolving a horrific event in the best way you can. It means integrating the trauma into your life in a way that now builds and strengthens you up when it once tore you apart. Recovery is accepting the unacceptable. It is acknowledging what you cannot change.

The Return to Joy and Innocence

There is a picture I hold in my mind from my work at a school, where a tragic shooting took the lives of some and injured many others. It is a memory I will hold for a lifetime.

I was asked to facilitate a professional debriefing group for students who had directly witnessed the shooting. After being assigned to particular classrooms, students, faculty, and families streamed down the usually active and bustling school hall in stunned silence.

I happened to glance at two young teenage girls whose images were forever recorded in my soul. With eyes glazed over from tears, they stared straight ahead to nowhere. Clasping each other's hand tightly, they moved past me as if in slow motion. My mind flashed for an instant to what they might have looked like the day before the tragedy. I imagined them with the expressions and exuberance normal to girls their age. I imagined their smiles and laughter. I thought about their conversations about after-school plans. I imagined for a moment my own daughter and her best friend walking in their shoes. And I saw the joy and innocence tragically stripped from their faces.

That morning, the joy and innocence was lost in hundreds of faces. I was to see the same scene over and over again in the weeks to come. They were different faces, but it was the same innocence, robbed of joy.

But joy was not permanently lost. In the weeks ahead, glimmers of it could be found on the faces of students when handed a new teddy bear, when hearing about the recovery of one of the wounded, or when being visited by the President of the United States—who offered personal words of comfort and consolation. Little by little, joy returned. Faces began to soften and relax. There was laughter in the halls again. Joy returned within the year for most, but for some it would take longer. For all, it was a sad day, never to be forgotten.

The love of family, friends, and skilled counselors will go a long way to heal your child. So will the simple passing of time. All are critical to your child's emotional repair process. However, whatever the trauma and loss you and your child have suffered, I believe it is through sharing a meaningful belief system and encouraging spiritual exploration that you can best help your child to heal.

As a concerned and loving parent, you have the opportunity to reconstruct a different view of the world than what your child has seen. Your child's heart is listening. Give voice to your love, and recovery will follow. It may feel like an extraordinary miracle, but life is full of them every day. On my way to work one morning, I read a quote on a billboard at a local car wash that said, "Nothing is as permanent as change." When something goes wrong, life seeks to right itself. Open wounds close, the winter makes way for spring, and life miraculously continues on in a constant state of renewal. Trauma means change, but so does healing.

Trauma has changed your child's life. Sorrow may linger and come again, but joy and innocence *will* return. The day will come when you may find yourself surprised by it or unexpectedly living in the midst of it. Or you may watch these feelings come back slowly in your child, like a long-awaited sunrise after a long, cold night. Either way, know that the return to joy and innocence is usually just around the bend.

Ways Adults Can Help— A Summary List

- Reestablish a sense of safety. Help children do whatever they need to in order to feel safe.

- Acknowledge the trauma/death honestly.

- Lessen demands.

- Lower expectations.

- Postpone any major decisions.

- Encourage normal routines and responsibilities.

- Maintain structure, but adjust for fears.

- Tolerate regression and feelings of anger.

- Talk about what happened.

- Encourage talk about thoughts and feelings.

- Educate and normalize thoughts and feelings.

- Model a way to express feelings openly.

- Talk about attitude changes and physical symptoms you notice and connect them to the trauma.

- Explain to children that the greater the loss, the longer it will take to heal.

- Give increased physical comfort and nurturing through special directed support.

- Reassure and share your hope for the future.
- Be patient and flexible.
- Share your confidence in your child's ability to heal.
- Indulge special needs.
- Identify positive memories that provide strength and humor during especially difficult times.
- Don't forget to have fun as a family.
- Be open to spiritual exploration.
- Let your children ask questions about their beliefs.
- Parent from a solid foundation of beliefs and values.
- Live your life in a way that teaches the value of life.
- Make a verbalized commitment to practice nonviolent behavior and language in your home.
- Take a stand and set limits around what you have control over such as exposure to violence in movies, music, books and television.
- Parent in a way that teaches by example.
- Reflect the standards and personal beliefs you hold through your parenting.

Remember:

- You cannot protect children or control what happens around them every minute of every day, even though you would like to.
- Troublesome behaviors are often expressions of feelings disguised.
- Acting out may be an effort to "numb out" or voice anger.
- There is always hurt under anger.
- Your child is not crazy—what happened was crazy.
- Seeking help is a sign of strength and an act of a loving parent.
- A balanced and healthy emotional life includes a spiritual foundation for your child.

🙋 Michael learned that hurricanes are not monsters and are not the result of anyone's anger but happen when the weather changes. He looked forward to drawing pictures of the storm in our sessions and planned ways he could feel prepared for another hurricane if one were to strike again. Michael enjoyed creating different endings to his nightmares by drawing me pictures of how he would block the wind from reaching people's homes. Michael and his dad studied hurricanes together and learned the facts about their formation and occurrence. He kept his new friend, "Freddie Jr.," hooked to a leash on his bed so that he would be able to find him easily if he had to leave quickly again. Michael told me hurricanes didn't scare him anymore because he knew it was just a "bunch of mixed-up weather that hardly ever happened." Both Amanda and Michael benefited from sleeping in the same room for a period of time and Michael's parents provided their children with more physical comfort through out the day and before bedtime. These measures helped Michael sleep more securely and his nightmares gradually diminished.

Amanda's parents stopped insisting she unpack her boxes. Instead they allowed her to keep her belongings however she wished. Amanda's mom even brought home some newer and stronger boxes with lids and a marker to label them to help her find things easier. They bought her a weather radio that she could tune into when she felt worried about the wind. A windsock on the fence outside her bedroom window helped her to monitor with a quick glance what was happening outside.

Amanda brought her best friend to one of our counseling sessions. They agreed that being together helped them feel better, so their parents found ways to help them spend more time together. They talked about their fears of a hurricane happening again. They created a plan for what they would do if it hit while they were at school and identified all the people and plans already in place that helped ensure their safety and the safety of the community.

Amanda looked forward to the new house her parents were having built on a different side of town. She decided she would "unpack" her boxes in the new house because it would feel safer. She told me she knew the hurricane could strike there too, though it was in an area that had survived this one well. Gradually, Amanda felt safe again and confidently moved on with her life.

After six months in counseling following the hurricane Amanda and her family survived, she said to me, "It's not that I want to leave you, but I don't really need you anymore. I really feel like myself again despite everything that's happened. My family has peace again."

🙋

Part II

How You Can Help: A Guide for Nonparental Adults

9

How Friends and Relatives Can Help

"You need nice families and friends. They can help you feel like yourself again."

Tracy was in the third grade when she was allowed to pick out her first dog. She chose an eight-week-old miniature Alaskan husky with puffy white fur. Tracy named him "Kuma," which in Japanese means "little bear."

Kuma and Tracy were fast friends and quickly bonded. Tracy was young to have the responsibility for training Kuma and caring for all the needs that come with a new puppy, but she learned quickly and eagerly with the help of her parents. Tracy took her responsibility seriously.

Kuma had been with Tracy only six weeks when a large neighborhood dog viciously attacked him. Before neighbors and parents were able to intervene, Kuma was killed. Tracy witnessed the attack and watched in horror as Kuma was savagely torn apart. They were the longest moments of her life.

Tracy told me later he was kissing her face just before he was attacked. She said, "He was in my arms all warm and happy one minute and the next thing I knew there he was . . . limp and pulled apart like an old stuffed animal. Only there was blood everywhere. When he stopped moving, I couldn't believe it was Kuma lying there and that he was really dead."

Tracy begged her parents to rush Kuma to the vet so they could operate and save him. She screamed frantically at them, "Daddy, hurry! Please! We've got to get him to the hospital! Let the doctors save him! They might be able to save him!" Tracy's father gently took hold of her shoulders and stooped down. Looking straight into her eyes he said, "Kuma is gone already Tracy. No one can save him. Kuma has died." Her father gently lifted her and when he did she fell limp into his arms and sobbed from a place so deep within that her whole body seemed to convulse in grief. A tidal wave of pain and heartbreak poured over her.

That night Tracy never stopped crying. She eventually fell asleep from exhaustion, but even when she woke, her eyes were still wet and streaming with tears. Everything she did and everywhere she looked reminded her of Kuma. But Tracy saw more in her mind than Kuma's food bowl, chew toys, and water dish. She was distressed by images of the attack and consumed by thoughts and feelings of helplessness and fear. She repeatedly heard the guttural growl of the attacking dog and the high pitched screams of her pup. Tracy's grief was complicated by the suddenness of the attack and the guilt she carried for not protecting Kuma or saving him in time. In her mind Tracy believed she had let Kuma be killed. She told me, "It's all my fault. I didn't stop the mean dog. I stood there and let him rip my Kuma up." Tracy had nightmares in which she relived the attack over and over. She stopped eating and became very sullen. "She's walking around like a robot," her mother told me.

Tracy's parents talked with her about the event. They comforted, consoled, and addressed her deepest worries. They told me, "Tracy is so sensitive that we really think this is going to continue to be very hard on her for some time." Her parents were right.

In addition to the loving presence of her parents, Tracy would soon discover great benefits from being in the presence of others who knew and loved her. When friends and relatives began to call and visit, the same love and comfort she experienced from her parents was given by others as well. It was during times of this additional support that Tracy's parents noticed she began to seem hopeful again.

One of Tracy's closest friends talked to her over the phone and listened to the whole story. It would be a story she would need to *tell again and again. Her friends, grandparents, aunts, uncles, and cousins let her tell the story to them as they listened eagerly and with undivided attention. Tracy especially liked it when she heard stories from others that had been through something like she had. Her granddad and uncle both told her about the losses they had experienced with a beloved pet. Her parents listened quietly as family members explained to Tracy why dogs sometimes attack each other and why she could never have intervened. With every story and every connection she had with others, her parents noticed that Tracy's face grew more relaxed and animated.*

Tracy's grandmother made a special frame for Tracy's favorite photo of Kuma. Together they colored pictures of him to hang in a special place in the house as a memorial to him. At dinner that night her uncle said grace and added in a prayer for Kuma and Tracy.

When I asked Tracy how the experience had changed her, she said, "It made me really scared and sad. And I found out it gets better after a while but not right away." I asked what had helped her the most to feel better, and she replied, "You need nice families and friends. They help you feel like yourself again."

Following a traumatic event, the very presence of trusted and loving friends and family members can help restore a sense of normalcy in children's lives. The security found in these relationships can add a rich sense of stability and support to a child's world. Children benefit from watching enduring relationships grow and deepen over time. They learn the value of supporting one another in times of celebration and sorrow. The connection you have with a traumatized child can be an important resource to his or her healing now.

Your Role in the Healing Process

If a child close to you has been impacted by a crime or trauma, you have been impacted, too. As a close friend or relative, it's common to feel upset and distressed as you stand by and see the child you care about changed by trauma. It may be difficult to hear about or see what your loved one survived.

Reading this book can be the first step in supporting the child you love. Educating yourself about the normal reactions children experience following a trauma will help you play an important role in their healing process.

It is natural to feel overwhelmed by a sense of helplessness. You may feel awkward, nervous, or unsure of how to approach the child and his or her immediate family. Friends and relatives want the opportunity to help, but often don't know how.

You may be struggling with questions like: What should I say? When should I help? Is it okay to ask about what happened? Should I try and be cheerful to make them feel better? How should I act around the children? Will I upset them if I say something about what happened? What if I cry? What can I do to take their pain away? It's a confusing time for everyone and it may feel hard, but this chapter can help you see that these difficult questions are really very easy to answer.

Listen and Ask

Traumatized children are forced into pain they weren't prepared for. If you can help them feel less alone and better understood, you can significantly change the course of their distress.

Listen to what your loved ones say they need and respect their wishes. When in doubt, just ask. Whether you are talking to children or their caregivers, your response can be guided by what they tell you. Be honest about your fears and concerns, and ask how you might be most helpful to them. Be direct and be yourself.

Say What You Feel

Here are some examples of how to say what you feel and express your true thoughts and feelings:

- I don't know what to say.
- I want so much to help, and I don't know how.
- I feel so many different emotions, I can only imagine what it must be like for you.
- I'm so sorry this has happened.
- I'm so sorry you are going through this.
- I'm so sorry you had to experience/hear about/see this.
- What can I do for you?
- Would you like to talk about what happened?
- Is this a good time to talk/come over?
- I want to hear about what you've been through when you'd like to tell me.

- I know no one can change what you've been through, but I want you to know I'm here in whatever way you need me, and I love you.

Ways to Assist

Be realistic:

- Don't act like it never happened.

- Unless you've been through similar life tragedies, it may be hard for you to understand what your loved ones are going through. If that's the case, be honest and say that.

- Recognize that no one can change what happened or take the pain away for another person.

- No matter how much you love and care for someone, you cannot stop the hurt. Love aids the healing process but it does not take it away. To try and "take away" children's pain minimizes the impact it had on them.

- Avoid using clichés that sound well-meaning but actually attempt to talk kids out of their true feelings, such as, "Let me see a great big smile," "There's always a rainbow after a storm," or "Put on a happy face."

- Don't change the subject or try and find the "good" in what happened. Well-meaning loved ones may mistakenly try and cheer up children and families who are in the midst of great pain. This will probably only to serve to alienate you from them.

- Be ready to assist and at the same time take care of yourself. Overextending yourself to help others, even people you love, will not help anyone.

Be supportive:

- Helping means being a good listener. Be sure you are listening more than you are talking.

- To comfort and console you must accept what it's like to be with your loved ones in their pain.

- Give alone time and respect their privacy when it's needed.

- Take food and healthy snacks.

- Send a card or note.

- In the months and years to come, remember to call or acknowledge the event in some way on days that will be reminders. For example, "I'm aware that today is the second anniversary of the trauma you suffered. How are you holding up?" and "Just wanted to let you know I'm thinking of you today. I know it may be a difficult one for you to get through because of _____ (be specific). How are you doing?" Speak (or write) directly about the event they survived or suffered. Don't be afraid to talk openly about memories of anyone who may have died. Calls and notes are often a welcomed interruption for those who didn't expect the significance of the day to be remembered by anyone.

Be available:

- Don't isolate or stay away from the child and his or her family.

- Be physically present when requested. Companionship is important.

- Be willing and available to be called on for assistance. Let your loved ones know they can ask you for what they need.

- Ask for specific ways you can help.

- Wait to give spiritual/religious consolation, unless asked. For now, just be with your friend or relative in their suffering.

Be a diversion. You can give primary caregivers a break. Offer to play with children and answer the questions that the parents may be weary of hearing. It can be especially helpful to plan special activities. The following list of ideas might help you think of some special ways to spend time with children who need you:

- Play cards or a board game.

- Work on a new puzzle together.

- Bring a special book to read together.

- Walk the dog together.

- Plant in a garden.

- Do a craft project.

- Cook together.

- Learn a new computer game.

- Bring stuffed animals, night-lights, or music tapes for them to enjoy.

Be an advocate:

- If a legal case is involved, help your loved ones find guidance through the criminal justice process.

- If you can, help the family financially if an event has imposed financial burdens on them. Assist them in securing appropriate medical or therapeutic care if needed.

Be respectful:

- Don't "hover" or be intrusive.

- Acknowledge the unique reactions of each person in the family.

- Let them grieve in their own way and in their own time frame.

- Refrain from making any judgments.

- Always gain permission from the parents before you contact the children. Ask them what would be most helpful or appreciated.

- Let children say no. Give them choices about your involvement and respectfully honor their decisions.

Be yourself:

- Be willing to laugh, cry, and share experiences on whatever level is genuine for you.

- Don't be afraid to be in a good mood, just be sensitive to why they may not be able to feel the same as you.

- Be yourself, even if you're happy. Let children be themselves, too. Don't hide or disguise your feelings unless they could be frightening for children to hear or see.

- Don't be afraid to share your memories, even humorous ones. It's okay as long as the children laugh with you.

- Don't be afraid to remember and talk openly about the trauma's impact and the loss that resulted.

Timing

You will need to determine when to step in and lend a hand and when to step back and give space. Timing and sensitivity are especially important right now.

Initially children may feel numb about what happened and appear to be coping well, when actually they are still in a state of shock. Don't mistake shock for strength. Children may not have experienced the full range of reactions when you see or visit them. It may not be until the shock wears off that you will see the full range of reactions appear. When that happens the work and pain begins. Children and their families may need your support *later* rather than sooner.

Remember, exhibiting symptoms and experiencing difficulties after a trauma is the normal reaction for healthy people to have. It is not a sign of strength or sound mental health to be *without symptoms*. To have reactions is to be healthy.

How Long Will It Take?

As a friend or family member, you might begin to feel impatient. You may wonder how long it takes before children affected by trauma can begin to feel better and act like "themselves" again. It is normal to want them to "hurry up and get better." It is also normal that they can't. Healing will take as much time as each child needs.

The chaos of trauma threatens to destroy the daily structure and routines an adult needs to maintain in order to uphold a job and family. The strain on relationships is usually significant. Help with household chores or yard work to relieve stress, and offer to take care of the day-to-day needs when you can. With emotional support and understanding, you will have assisted your loved ones in ways that can help restore emotional balance and stability.

How Siblings Are Affected

Having brothers and sisters can help children feel less alone in the world. Sibling relationships can be one of the most constant and lasting connections a child can have. After a trauma, sibling relationships can change significantly in ways that can both help and hamper the recovery process.

Trauma can produce added strain on sibling relationships. Feelings about one another may change. A six-year-old girl told me that ever since her older brother had witnessed a gang shooting, "he was no fun anymore." She said, "He doesn't like to play with me. I hate him now." Siblings can feel frightened and worried about the changes they see in their brothers or sisters. Feelings of insecurity are evoked when any previously secure relationship is disrupted. Siblings may fight more and act out from fear and anxiety. Jealousy may also erupt if all the attention from others is focused on the child most impacted.

When siblings are bonded in helpful ways, they can be instrumental to each other through the healing process. Sometimes siblings can be an added source of strength to one another, especially at times when parents are not as available to them.

Anna and Emily were a source of comfort and companionship for each other after they witnessed a physical attack on their parents. They slept together for a period of time and invented a storytelling game that helped them fall asleep at night. They came to my office together one week and Anna, the older sister, was tearful. She told me they had argued through the bathroom door that morning and she had yelled, "Get out! I was ahead!" Anna explained she was angry because she was supposed to get the bathroom first. Emily thought she heard, "I wish you were dead." She bolted out of the bathroom and ran to her room sobbing, deeply hurt by her sister's words. Once Anna figured out what happened, she explained the misunderstanding and repeatedly apologized and reassured her sister that she could never even think such a thing.

As Anna relayed the incident to me, she welled up in tears and explained how much she loved her sister. She told Emily directly, "I love you, I would never *wish on you what almost happened to Mom and Dad."*

How You Can Help Siblings

When one child in a family has been impacted by trauma more severely than others, parental attention may be diverted for a while. Friends and relatives can help by seeking opportunities to attend to the children less directly affected.

You can help children understand the normal reactions they might expect to see in their brother or sister since the trauma. Prepare them for the different ways they might think and feel for a while. Help them understand the time it will take for their sister or brother to feel like themselves again. Explain that they may be intensely sensitive to comments others make about what happened or about the way they are reacting. Help them understand this is natural. Let them know they can talk to you if they need help or grow frustrated with their brother or sister. Support the siblings' responses and help them realize that *their* feelings are normal too.

It will be important to help siblings understand why they can expect to see many people rally around their brother or sister with attention. You can explain that it is right and fair that their brother or sister be given extra help and support at this time, just as anyone in the family would with a physical illness. One uncle explained it to his nephew by saying, "It's your brother's turn to get help from your mom and dad right now. When you or I need extra help, then we'll get it, too. Families take turns being there for each other. Our job right now is to help out in other ways and to be understanding. You and I can do that together."

When you can, give every child a role in the healing process. Help siblings think of ways they can help and make a contribution to their brother or sister's well-being. Find plenty of ways to acknowledge them directly for their helpfulness and resourcefulness. Help them find time away from the situation if that's needed.

Check out the reactions of every child in the family. Sometimes the kids who appear to be fine and unaffected are in fact struggling internally. Pay close attention to each child, and when you can, equally spread your affection and comfort around.

Talk openly to children, together and separately, about what's going on for each of them. Remind them it is normal to have many different feelings at once. Remember that they are different people with their own perceptions and experiences. Honor the feelings unique to each one.

How Grandparents Can Help

If you're a grandparent, you may be more important than you know. If you have a special relationship with your grandchildren, you can be instrumental in helping them find resiliency in the midst of despair and difficulties. How do you know if your relationship is special enough to do that? Answer the following three questions: Do you enjoy playing with your grandchild? Do you laugh often and loudly together? Do you have fun while you're together?

If you answered yes to one, you probably answered yes to all three. Congratulations. You are a source of natural healing for your grandchild. If you answered no to these questions, take the steps to change the answer to just one and your relationship will be a new source of healing for your grandchild.

When children are fortunate enough to know their grandparents, their relationship can add another dimension to their lives, to their families, to their sense of belonging in the world, and to their healing from trauma.

Giving

As a grandparent, you may be especially revered for what surprises you bring to your grandchildren. After a tragedy, children may be less enthusiastic about anything you give them, but bring your ideas anyway. They can be healing. While gifts of monetary value are often appreciated, they are by no means the only way to your grandchild's heart. Things that are meaningful to you can be just as meaningful to them. Try some of the following ideas when you visit next:

- Bring materials for handmade gifts or crafts you can work on together.
- Brush or style your grandchild's hair.
- Share a special recipe you can make together.
- Take your grandchild out for an ice cream cone.
- Help them start a collection of something, such as stickers, buttons, baseball cards, or stamps.
- Give your grandchild old photos of you and/or his or her parents.
- Pass down something of sentimental value, such as an old ring, a doll from your childhood, or a family tree.
- Give soaps or the pen and stationary you collected from your last hotel room.
- Give things from nature that you find where you live, such as pine cones, sea shells, rocks, autumn leaves, or pressed flowers from your yard.

When they come from grandparents, every gift can be a treasure. Giving things of meaning can be an expression of your love.

Kids Deserve to Be Treated Like They're Special

After trauma, children need to feel important again for who they are, not just for what they've been through. Your attention can help them feel special again and build self-esteem. You can do the important job of reminding children how truly special they are. When you do not live with your grandchildren, you are probably more likely to appreciate every moment you have with them. If you do live with your grandchildren, your influence on their development can be a special gift. Whatever your situation, the excitement you share about wanting to be with them can be healing.

Give Kids a Break

Just like parents need a break from the role of parenting, kids need a break from the way they're parented. Following the stress of trauma, grandparents can provide needed relief to both children and parents alike. Grandparents who visit from out of town provide a distraction for children from regular routines and schedules. A visit from you can be like taking a mental vacation for your grandchildren. Though it's temporary, kids may get to loosen up and do things they may not normally get to do every day. This is good for everyone. Flexibility and change in a family benefits all.

The other powerful role you can play is that of being a good listener and companion. If you have the luxury to give more undivided attention to your grandchildren than other adults, you may notice and observe something parents are too close to see or hear. Your grandchildren may be able to say things to you about their experience that they are unable to say to their parents or anyone else. Sometimes advice can come easier from you, too.

You have wisdom to share, so share it and enrich your grandchildren's lives in the process. Here is a short sampling of what you have to offer them in the aftermath of a tragedy:

- You can draw from your many years of parenting experience.

- You can choose to react less and listen more.

- You can teach what you know about tragedy, life and loss.

- You can be an example of a survivor.

- You can build healthy self-esteem.

- You can be the refuge in a storm.

- You can be a source of strength.

- You can share your beliefs and values.

- You can tell great stories about your grandchildren's parents and your own life in the "olden days."

- You can be an advocate for your grandchildren.

- You can be their biggest fan.

- You can be their best audience.

- You can teach about the natural life process of aging.

- You can protect.

- You can soothe and comfort.

- You can be a reservoir of love.

You can be all these things and more if you choose.

Don't be afraid to talk openly about the trauma that has touched all of your lives. Be willing and available to let grandchildren talk and tell you all about what's on their minds. Or allow them to be with you for relief and to have a break from talking about the trauma. You may be the only one who can help them forget about it for a while. Both roles are of equal value to your grandchild in the healing process.

Stay Connected

If you enjoy and look forward to time with your grandchild, you have all that it takes to help them. If you live out of town, you can still have a powerful presence in their lives. Letters, cards, audio tapes, video recordings, photos, stories, postcards, pictures, or a box of fudge or cookies can light up an otherwise gloomy day.

My daughter received a special surprise in the mail from her grandparents shortly after they learned she had lost many of her favorite belongings when our home was burglarized. She carefully sifted through a box of homemade treats and found a small but heavy foil wrapped packet with her name on it. She opened it excitedly, certain it was her favorite chocolate chip cookies or a new piggy bank to replace the one the intruders had broken. She looked confused when liquid dripped down her fingers.

She was shocked and amused to find a used slab of old lunch meat inside. It had a green glow. "Uh-oh," she said, "I think Grams and Gramps have finally lost it." A quick phone call confirmed the mistake and this story continues to be one of my daughter's favorites. She promises to tease them forever about the slimy meat they accidentally sent to try and cheer her up. Nevertheless, it did cheer her up. The special belongings that were stolen or damaged represented a heartfelt loss, but the slimy green meat lifted the seriousness of it all. Clearly, her relationship with her grandparents was far more valuable than a new piggy bank.

No matter what you give or send, make the effort to stay connected to your grandchildren. The fact that you are involved in their lives can mean a lot. When you do stay connected, you can be one of the most profound factors in their recovery.

10

For Teachers and Professional Therapists

"Thank you for helping me get my family back."

In our last session, nine-year-old Miguel gave me a thank-you card that read, "Thank you for helping me get my family back." His acknowledgment and awareness of what he had lost, as well as what he gained back, provided us with rich discussion for our last session. His card provided the closure we needed for our work together to be complete.

Guidelines for Teachers

Trauma symptoms prevent children from performing at their usual level in school. They may feel tired and find it difficult to pay attention. Their concentration may be continually disrupted by distressing internal and external stimuli. Children often feel inpatient with themselves for not being able to act like they used to. If they experience more pressure from school, they are likely to fall further behind in their studies.

You can help rebuild academic confidence in students by reassuring them that their reactions are normal. Help kids know that you and others will help them cope with the tasks and requirements they face. Keep your expectations realistic and simple. Every child will be different.

Please note: In addition to this section for teachers, please refer to "School Life" in chapter 2. The information and suggestions given to parents will be beneficial for you to know and can increase the possibility for successful collaboration.

Acknowledge and Adjust

Ignoring trauma in the life of students will not prevent them from thinking about it or help make it any less difficult. It is important to recognize the event and appropriately accommodate the reactions you see exhibited. There are general guidelines to keep in mind as you approach and work with students who have been impacted by a trauma:

- *Directly acknowledge the trauma to your student.* You might say something like, "What you've been through has been tough," "I'm so sorry it happened, and I'm glad you're okay," "How can I help on your first day back to school?" and/or "We can do some things differently for a while until you feel like yourself again."

- *Stay in close contact with parents or guardians.* Find out what concerns or special needs they have identified that can help you work better with the child. Listen to their ideas about what approach they think will be helpful to use with their child. Share your thoughts and impressions and ask for their feedback. Follow up regularly on what may or may not be working. Request permission from parents to consult with professional counselors the child is seeing (if applicable). Working together, you can create a unified base of support for your student and increase the likelihood of a successful transition back to school.

- *Respond and adjust to increased fears and feelings of insecurity.* It will be helpful to maintain the usual structure and routine that students are used to. If children are worried about family members while at school, come up with a plan to help. For instance, you might devise a time where children call home or receive notes of encouragement from loved ones throughout the day.

- *Be sensitive to peer group relations and reactions from friends.* Some teachers find it helpful to encourage classroom discussions about ways friends can support and respect one another after one or more of the children has been through a difficult experience.

- *Let children complete homework and school work at their own pace.* Ask them which assignments or worksheets they will be able to complete and what they need to back off from for now. With their help, determine how much they can realistically accomplish each day. Reassure them that as time goes by they will be able to keep up with their work again.

- *Encourage office staff to keep track of physical symptoms.* When children visit the office with health complaints, encourage the school nurse or office personnel to document illnesses. Chronic headaches or stomach upsets may signal continued distress that will require more help by a professional therapist and/or physician. This information will be important to pass on to other caretakers involved in the student's life.

When Trauma Touches Everyone in Your Class or School

Imagine for a moment that one of the following scenarios has taken place:

Just as they are arriving one morning, children witness a car accident in front of your school. A fellow student is struck on his bike, thrown thirty feet into the middle of the road, where he remains, unconscious.

As school lets out one afternoon, children watch helplessly as a parent begins battering his partner, hitting her on the head with a lead pipe. She is thrown to the ground, screaming, surrounded by a pool of blood.

What would you say to your students after such a tragedy occurred? Teachers often tell me they are afraid they will "say the wrong thing" or upset their students more by mentioning the incident.

When a situation has touched the lives of everyone in your class, the need to talk about what happened is real. Don't be afraid to discuss what happened. Kids need to vent and hear that others feel like they do, and they need the opportunity to receive accurate information. Discuss the event in simple, factual, and honest terms. Take time to listen to students' ideas and theories and correct any misunderstandings to help prevent the spread of unfounded rumors. Safety issues will also need to be addressed to calm children's fears and worries.

Uncertainties are a part of life. As a teacher, you have the perfect opportunity to teach your students an important lesson: You can help children learn how to live through the experience of fear, grief, and sorrow within a supportive group setting. Help kids to experience your classroom as an understanding environment. When children are tearful, remind them that letting out tears when they feel sad is one way to help themselves feel better. Make your classroom a place where kids can find support and companionship. There is comfort in participating in routine tasks and existing in a predictable structure. Both contribute to reestablishing a sense of security and relaxation, which are critical components to being in the right frame of mind for learning.

Classroom Activities That Can Help

Allowing children to work through an event together can enable them to resume their normal daily schedules with less distress and distractions. You may want to incorporate some of the following activities to help students come to terms with a trauma:

- Discuss the facts of the trauma as if writing a newspaper article. List on the board the who, what, where, when, and how of what happened. Be factual, forthright, and honest, without sharing graphic details that can add to a child's anxiety.

- Focus on the resolution of the event. What was handled well? Identify who or what helped the situation. Who was most helpful? List all the good things that people did in the aftermath. This activity can help control fears children may have about the tragedy happening again.

- Talk about different reactions to the event. Make lists for each of the following categories: Heart (feelings), Mind (thoughts), Body (physical symptoms), Soul (meaning, questions, beliefs). Encourage children to think about ways they have been affected in each area. Acknowledge that what happened can be sad and frightening for everyone. As children share their reactions, ask, "Do others feel the same way?" and "How is it different or the same for you?"

- Use open-ended phrases and fill in the blank completion sentences. These exercises may help students identify some of their reactions. Here are some examples:

I feel _____ because _____ .

I think about _____ when _____ .

I wonder about _____ because _____ .

I (do what) _____ when I feel _____ .

I can talk to _____ about my thoughts and feelings.

- Make a confidential question box that children can put their questions into whenever they want to. Spend time each day answering some of the questions together as a class. Some teachers of older students have each student take a question, research some solutions, and then write an "advice column." They can be posted around the room and discussed.

- Create a project where small groups of students design a poster about one aspect of healing, such as the heart, mind, body, or soul. For example, one group could research ways to cope with difficult feelings and emotions (the heart). Have students list helpful suggestions and coping tools on these posters, which can be displayed throughout the school.

- Allow children time to draw pictures or write notes, poems, songs, stories, or letters to express their feelings and offer condolences to victims. Help them find ways to satisfy their desire to help.

- Invite guest speakers to come in and share information that might help build feelings of confidence and security.

- Create a class project during which children put together first-aid kits for their homes and classrooms.

Make Your Class a "Trauma-free Zone"

Be careful not to expose your class to unnecessary information or to traumas in progress via the television, radio, or adult conversations in your classroom.

I received a call from someone who was concerned about a first-grade class at her school whose teacher had turned on the television in her room to watch a tragedy unfold at another local school. The caller appropriately questioned the judgment of this action and the potential impact it may have had on the children in the class, even though they did not appear to be watching it themselves.

It was not surprising to learn that parents called the following day complaining that their children had come home frightened and worried about the news program they had listened to at school. Some children feared for the safety of their siblings at different schools and others believed the trauma had actually happened at their school and didn't want to return the following day. Even though they appeared to be involved and concentrating elsewhere, the television reports were frightening and confusing to many of the students.

Children who have histories of trauma may be particularly vulnerable and sensitive to any stimuli of this kind. Be a buffer between your students and disturbing information when you can. Children are never too young to be affected by what's going on around them, and young children will be developmentally incapable of making sense of it.

When Humor Is Uncomfortable

Some teachers are dismayed or angered when students minimize or make jokes about a traumatic event. I am often asked how teachers should respond to such situations. It is important to openly acknowledge the feelings you observe and remind students of the many forms pain can take. Talk about some of the responses uncomfortable feelings can evoke in people. You also might want to say something like "Sometimes it's easier to laugh than cry," "Pain can be expressed in many different ways," "Jokes might help you and others better cope with what happened," "However you choose to cope, it's important to be respectful here," and/or "Don't be surprised if jokes stop feeling funny. Eventually everyone must face their pain."

Be Prepared

Returning to a "normal" school day routine as soon as possible after a tragedy can be reassuring to kids. But remember, the days following a trauma are anything but normal. A "normal" day does not mean using denial or becoming rigid in your plans for the day. It means sticking to a routine the best you can while openly acknowledging and adjusting to what's different. This will be true for anniversary dates of the trauma as well.

Your students will be watching and observing your responses to traumatic news and discussions. Be calm and undramatic. Before attending to your pupils be sure that you and all school staff involved have been able to receive group debriefings *separate from the children.* Before you can be there for your students, be sure someone is there for you, too. Don't hesitate to ask for help in the task of facilitating discussions if what happened has personally hit too close to home.

Ask that someone trained to assist children with post-traumatic stress be assigned to assist you or help you lead a classroom discussion. Do what you can, even if that means modeling for your class the strength it takes to seek help and support.

Strengthen School Environments with a Customer Service Mentality

What happens to kids when they walk into your school each morning? If every child who came through the door was treated like your best "customer," chances are your school environment would change.

Wally Bryant is a principal at an elementary school in Eugene, Oregon. Every morning (many of which are dripping wet), Wally stands at the entrance to his school and personally greets every child that walks past him. He smiles, acknowledges students by name, wishes them a good morning, gives a pat on the back now and then, and has a good laugh every so often. Wally even helps students get out of their cars when parents have their hands full. He wears fun ties every day, his school T-shirt on school spirit days, and outrageous costumes for the annual carnival. Wally's staff know kids by their first names, too. Every year at the school talent show, Wally and his staff perform a comedy act that "brings the house down." Despite his shy demeanor, Wally has even been known to don a tutu on center stage. He does it all for the kids he serves.

Wally and other staff like him understand what it means to have a "service" mentality. His first job is to help every student feel welcome and valued. Students need to feel cared for and loved. When they are, success in school increases.

School teachers, administration, and staff members have the opportunity to create a family atmosphere on their campus without compromising high standards of academic and behavioral excellence. And a supportive environment is the first step to helping your school stay safe. It also helps students build resiliency to stress. If trauma should strike in such an atmosphere, students will be further along on the road to healing because of the nurturing environment around them.

Look around your school. Is every child being treated as if they were your best "customer"? If not, make a commitment to serve the kids you work for and encourage your school to adopt a customer service mentality. It will go a long way in helping school environments become happier, healthier, and safer.

What Professional Therapists Need to Know

Trauma work requires training and preparation. Mental health counselors and therapists need to take several professional and personal roads before entering this field. Personal preparation and professional training are required before your work can successfully begin.

A Heart for Trauma: Personal Preparation

Do you have a heart for trauma? Many professionals work in this field for personal reasons. You don't have to be a survivor of trauma yourself to be useful and effective, but it helps. You may not have experienced exactly what your client has, but if you've survived a trauma you know the process of healing because you've lived through it. You can be living proof that healing happens.

It is imperative that you successfully resolve any and all trauma in your life before you attempt to help others. If you don't have a handle on the experience of coping and healing from post-traumatic stress, don't fake it. The kids will know.

The Decision to Work with Kids and Trauma

I never planned on being a child therapist. At one point, I would have thought I had as much chance of working with kids as I had of becoming a rocket scientist. I never would have believed that I would grow into a career working with children, let alone those who had witnessed homicides and other violent crimes. I would have thought that the idea was utterly impossible and far too difficult a responsibility for me to handle. But when I was asked to work in this field, I had only to look as far as my daughter to make my decision. I asked myself one question, "What kind of help and attention would I want my daughter to receive if this crime had happened in front of her?" More people are needed to attend to this growing population. It was too important to refuse.

I learned that while trauma conditions are despicable, the children and the work helping them recover is deeply satisfying. If you enter this field, you will receive more than you can ever give back. Therein lies the joy in trauma work.

The decision to work with children impacted by trauma is a serious choice. It's not for everyone. Children must feel safe, protected, and able to confide in you their deepest feelings, fears, doubts, guilt, and questions. You must be able to hear disturbing details and sometimes grisly descriptions. Children need to know their thoughts and feelings won't worry or frighten you and that you can hear it all. They need to see that you can handle whatever they need to say.

No matter how much you already love kids, not all skilled and compassionate therapists can bear witness to such unspeakable crimes. In order to be effective, you must have a heart for this work and receive specialized training to learn how to bring your heart wisely into your work.

Your Role with Parents

There is no substitute for family and parent involvement in a child's healing process. Working with children changed by trauma will require that you provide parent education and support to caretakers. You don't have to be a parent to do that well, but it helps. You will need to be comfortable and competent employing parent education strategies that empower parents to take an active role in their child's recovery.

Throughout your work, maintain open communication with parents and at the same time respect the privacy of the children who are your clients. Children need to know that you will hold what they say and do confidential unless it's a safety concern. Clearly communicate your therapeutic boundaries and ethical standards to both adults and children so everyone knows what to expect.

Parents hold a position you can't and shouldn't duplicate. They are in the position to supply the greatest love, security, and guidance possible for children and do it on a twenty-four-hour basis. But in the midst of trauma, caretakers often need your help to know where and how to begin.

A Mind for Trauma: Professional Training

You can't receive all the professional training you will need from books and classroom experience alone. Along with the educational pieces, you will need to find trained colleagues or supervisors who can mentor and guide you through practical experiences.

Training and experience in play and art therapy is essential to working with traumatized children. Marriage and family counseling training will also be invaluable as you help families navigate their way through parenting challenges and added stress that may be present in all their relationships. You will need to know when and how to incorporate multiple modalities of treatment with individuals, families, siblings, parents, couples, and peer support groups.

Homicide Requires Even More Training

Homicide survivors present an even greater training challenge because the issues are so complex and multifaceted. Grieving the loss of someone who has been killed suddenly, violently, and senselessly is different from any other form of grieving. It's something that everyone is unprepared for. The anguish is intense and long-lasting. Sometimes the pain is too deep for words. Images of the death or knowledge of a loved one's last moments may be overwhelming. The physical and emotional reactions to the trauma are only the beginning. Criminal justice systems, insurance companies, settlements, and media can present a multitude of frustrations for families and their children and often repeatedly cause a return to initial trauma reactions.

Blending Skills with Intuition

Like nurturing parents, skilled clinicians will be able to integrate a sense of genuine empathy, respect, and hope into their work. Compassion is healing in and of itself, but to do this work well, seek training in all phases of trauma intervention and theory.

Two important roles you will provide through your work is that of caregiver and educator. These dual roles require you to use both skills and intuition. You will need to know when and how to utilize specific trauma-related interventions that are important to successful trauma resolution. You will need to be familiar with therapeutic techniques that counteract feelings of helplessness and encourage active coping and increased confidence. At times you will be challenged to create effective interventions on the spot.

When to Change the Rules

Initial assessments need to be thorough and comprehensive. In-depth information needs to be obtained about the child's and family's past history of trauma and coping skills. Family assessments will be necessary to determine current strengths and weaknesses of family communication and relational skills.

Working with children and their families in the acute stages of trauma sometimes requires the flexibility and wisdom to change the rules. Often, initial meetings will need to be longer. Clients must feel free to tell their story without being stopped midway through. One parent told me that as her adolescent son told his story to his counselor for the first time, the counselor encouraged him to keep expressing the experience along with his deepest emotions. Then the counselor suddenly said, "Time's up. You need to learn how to come out of it." The client left with information and images dredged up that had no place to go. While therapeutic limits are valuable and session time can be important to adhere to, the initial sessions of trauma work require time, care, and caution. It is important to pace and allow plenty of support as children move through their stories. To do otherwise is to do a serious disservice to your client, and it could prove to traumatize them further.

Cultural and Spiritual Awareness

A person's faith or belief system is personal and intimate. Take the time to increase your knowledge and understanding of cultures and/or religions different from your own. Family values and standards may differ depending on the culture or beliefs of each family. Make sure your waiting room and therapy playroom are filled with toys, books, and reading materials that reflect the diversity of the kids you are serving. They will feel more comfortable if there are toys that look like them and reflect their families.

In order to openly address and respond to spiritual exploration, it is helpful to have your own belief system intact. To work in this field it will help to have your own firm foundation from which to operate. It can be a stabilizing influence and springboard for your own self-support. If you aren't comfortable exploring spiritual issues, consider referring families to clergy or other spiritual counselors who can address these concerns with them.

When Trauma Hurts a School or Community

After a wide-scale tragedy, kids and their families need to gather together. If you've received training and have experience in critical incident debriefing you know the value and benefits for those who choose to participate. Critical incident debriefing is one of the clinical terms used to describe the process of bringing traumatized people together to begin talking about what happened. The process is structured, it has a time limit, and it serves to normalize reactions, provide tools, and help integrate painful memories. Participants are usually relieved to be able to share their experiences with others who went through what they did. It is not psychotherapy. The groups are small, voluntary, and confidential. Educational information and written lists of referrals for ongoing help and crisis intervention are distributed.

Though it may sound simple, facilitating critical incident debriefing groups requires special training and experience to ensure a positive and advantageous experience for participants.

On-site Etiquette and Respect

If you are asked to go to the site of trauma to offer assistance, use caution and discretion. Professionals who are called in are usually strangers in the midst of a close and connected group of children and their families. Treat schools or other groups you are assisting like you would a family you were seeing for the first time in treatment. Respect the school's needs in the same way you would respect a family's needs. Give schools or other groups the necessary time and space to come to grips with what they've been through.

Respect the variety of needs traumatized children and the adults around them will have. In your eagerness to assist and help kids vent, you may unknowingly infringe on their personal space and privacy. Your presence may be seen as intrusive rather than helpful. Build relationships with people first. Stay in the background and respect that kids and families will seek you out if and when they need you.

In the case of a school shooting where I was asked to assist on site, I chose to visit the library every week and met casually with people. Informally and without therapeutic intention, I simply sat, listened, and empathized. I got to know people so they could learn of options without feeling the potential pressure or stigma of needing a therapist. Reactions to trauma are not a sign of weakness, but the public you deal with may connect your presence with being "crazy." Trauma makes you feel crazy enough. Don't descend on survivors as if they need to seek your help. Build relationships and be of service, but don't impose your professional expertise on anyone who doesn't need or want it.

Children in the Middle

Some children are in the difficult position of living between two worlds. They are the children who are victims of a trauma and have a relationship with the person who is to blame for the trauma. In one world they share the grief, horror, loss, and traumatic reminders of an alarming event. In the other world, they grieve and experience the horror and fear for the friend or relative who caused the traumatic event.

A young girl who was severely traumatized by a drive-by shooting she witnessed learned that the gunman was her older cousin who she shared a close relationship with. Kids who are struggling with their own reactions to a trauma and at the same time feel loyalty to whoever is to blame for what happened are impacted two times. First there is the trauma of hearing about or experiencing the event. Then, there is the trauma of hearing the person responsible for the tragedy is someone you know and love. The world falls apart twice.

When children discover a friend or loved one has perpetrated unspeakable crimes, they may hold feelings of anger and hate directed at the person's deeds and behaviors, but they may simultaneously hold feelings of love from the bonds that have previously formed. The incongruency of these feelings is confusing to live with and can generate public outrage from those who are unable to tolerate any show of support for those who have caused a tragedy.

A student was convicted of driving under the influence after crashing his car into another vehicle and seriously injuring three of its passengers. The drunk driver's younger sister was close friends with two of the injured passengers in the car he struck. She was outraged, angry, and in distress for her injured friends, and at the same time she felt sorry for her brother, who had made a terrible mistake. Her loyalty and reactions to the perpetrator were mixed. She did not know whether to love or hate him. She felt both ways but didn't feel either reaction was right. She was ostracized and shamed for supporting her brother, but found it impossible to turn completely against him.

These children need a personal therapist who can support them through the long-term work of accepting both sides of the love/hate dilemma. Therapeutic concerns include helping children learn how to resolve feelings of guilt and responsibility for their loved one's actions. They may also feel it is their job to make amends to all the victims involved or to defend the loved one to whom anger is being directed. Children need to be told they can't rescue or change the offender, no matter how close they were or how much they love that person. Help children stabilize their torn emotions by reminding them of the reality of the situation: the offender(s) must be held accountable for his or her actions in the same way all people would after committing a crime or making a choice that ended up hurting someone. All of these issues prevent them from being able to discern their own reactions from those of others. Help them take care of troubling symptoms and allow their own personal grieving response to unfold in their own time.

The loss and impact for children who are torn between a personally traumatic experience and a relationship with the person who is the cause of their pain and suffering is nothing less than tumultuous. They deserve the same care, respect, and attention that any survivor and victim would receive, if not more.

When Your Work is Done

Part of your job is to help children believe that when it's all over and done, life is still worth living, even when part of it is beyond their control. Your goals will be to rebuild security, hope, and meaning. Help children depend on you for as long as they need, and at the same time help them leave you confidently as soon as their work is done.

One way to determine whether or not clients are getting better is to simply ask them. From the beginning sessions through to the end, you might ask questions like:

- What feels better?
- What feels worse?
- What's different for you since it happened?
- What's the same?
- What is your greatest fear right now?
- What was your greatest fear before?
- What are you doing that helps you cope?
- How will you know when you are better / have achieved emotional balance again?
- What will your life look like when you're done with counseling?
- What will you be doing?
- How will you know when it's time to stop counseling?
- How do you imagine you'll be coping when you're ready to stop?

Children exhibit a range of behaviors when healing has progressed to the point of being ready to end their work with you. Children may return to normal levels of energy, feel free of pain and distress, experience play as "fun" again, increase their experiences of pleasure, feel excited about the future and coming events, hold a sense of hopefulness in general, and participate freely with their friends and peer groups.

Children are ready to move forward when they are coping well, have reached an understanding of the trauma, and have found acceptance or meaning through the process of healing.

The Importance of a Positive Ending

Traumatized children have suffered an event with an unhappy ending. It is important to transition children and families through their ending with you in a confident and caring way. When children leave therapy because they've been empowered to leave and they understand why they're leaving and have expressed to you what their thoughts and feelings around this choice are, then you have provided a positive experience of ending a relationship in a healthy way. Plan and prepare ahead of time for a special ending session. Involve your clients in the creation of a meaningful last experience for them. Sometimes planning the last session can be made easier knowing you have an "open door policy" to therapy. Encourage your clients to return for a check-in session at a mutually agreed upon time or at any point if new concerns or challenges emerge.

Saying Good-bye

If it's hard for children to let go and say good-bye to you, help them put their feelings into words and normalize the experience as a natural and human consequence to any loss. At the same time you can share the confidence you hold in their abilities to move on without you. If *you* can't let go, this is an issue for supervision. Holding on to clients when it is not in *their* best interest can result in a destructive end to all your work together.

What to Do with Gifts

Most professionals have clearly stated ethical policies around receiving, giving, or exchanging gifts with clients. There are important reasons for setting limits around this and other boundary issues. However, children love to give gifts and sometimes it's the only way they know how to say good-bye. Many will spend much time and precious thought to giving you a small token of their appreciation. They may make you a card, draw you a picture, or write you a thank-you note. Children need to be free to give and find ways to put words and meaning to their acts of giving. You might encourage this by asking questions like, "If your gift could talk, what would it say to me?" "How could you express what you feel without your gift?" and/or "What can your gift say that you can't?"

Ways You Might Respond to Giving

What you might say: "I will treasure what you made for me because it is a part of you," "Even though I could never forget you, this picture will always remind me of your time here and our work together," and/or "Your words to me are as special as your gift."

Taking Care of Yourself

Do not attempt to work with children and trauma without a secure and reliable support system for yourself. You will need to know how to grieve in healthy ways, use humor to balance your perspectives, and possess a steadfast belief in the possibility for healing.

You will need to approach the work with your own emotional equilibrium in tact. It will help if your own foundation of beliefs is solid and firm. The meaning you find in life can help others find theirs.

"Debriefing" yourself is essential. Taking in traumatic material on a regular basis can be like drinking low doses of toxic poison. Unless you know what psychic antidotes you can use to remedy it, the ongoing exposure could prove professionally lethal. You need to know how to take care of yourself and eliminate the effects of what you will be exposed to.

If you have children, be careful about what you bring home. Secondary trauma reactions can affect your family when they hear phone consults or see pictures or read information about what you are doing. Answer questions in general terms that help your children understand the positive ways you are working with others to help them heal.

Activities to Soothe the Heart, Mind, Body, and Soul

Like the children you're treating, it is important to attend to your feelings, thoughts, physical care, and spiritual needs when working in the field or responding to traumatized children. What are some ways you can attend to your own heart, mind, body, and soul? Write up a list and post it somewhere to remind yourself to actively engage in activities in each of these areas. Don't forget the power of humor to balance pain and stress.

Here are some suggestions: spend time with the one who knows you best, listen to music, pray or meditate, write, walk, clean, read, ride a horse or bike, bake, create art, go to a sporting event, watch your favorite movie, attend a place of spiritual retreat, hike in the woods, visit a river or ocean, canoe on a lake, have fun with your kids, and/or seek out supervision or consultation.

Finally, remember your purpose for why you do what you do, and why you'll do it again.

Epilogue

I wrote most of this book ten years ago even though the words never found their way to paper. I carried it around in my mind, thinking that if I waited long enough, the need for it would be obsolete. In that time I moved from big cities to smaller communities thinking my work (and the need for it) would change significantly. But the truth is, now children are exposed more to trauma, not less. And where you live has nothing to do with it.

The good news is when caring adults invest quantities of quality time in the lives of children, good things happen. Trauma changes you, but love holds the power to change trauma. Your relationship with your children is the most important one they have, even when they are old enough to say it isn't. It is through your relationship with your children that they can discover resiliency, hope, and healing.

It's true that children who swim through a steady stream of tragedy must have extraordinary coping skills. They cannot avoid or deny their pain without serious consequences. Having read this book, my hope is that you are better equipped and encouraged to help children cross the paths of a sometimes dangerous and unpredictable world—with new skills to assist them as they make the journey. Be ready to walk with them through their adversity and struggles. You can show them that strength and endurance can prevail in time of need. Even in the worst of life situations your words can restore hope.

A friend and colleague once asked me, "What was the one thing you needed the most after your trauma?" A flurry of ideas raced through my mind as I searched for the one most important answer. I found it still sitting inside me as strong and clear as the day I first discovered it. *What I needed most was to be understood. I wanted others to grasp the life-altering experience the trauma had been for me.* I wanted others to know, not just because I needed to say it, but because I believed people needed to hear it. For me, it was headline news.

But like many traumas people endure, the car crash I survived was hardly noticed by anyone. It didn't make headlines or even the back page of the local newspaper. It was an explosion of glass and metal that happened silently in the midst of the day-to-day events that did make news that day. It happened quietly behind the scenes of a busy bustling world. But in my world it was the most profound, life-altering experience I had ever known.

I had many sympathetic listeners, but few people, I felt, really understood how the trauma had changed me. In the aftermath of my experience, it wasn't just the memories of crashing glass and metal that filled my mind with noise. It was the silence of those not listening that was deafening. And it was the quiet loss of safety, the stillness of facing death, that I kept hearing. But despite all the physical and emotional anguish, it was also a time that proved to me that hope can be born out of chaos. It was the bend in the road that permanently changed my life view in a positive way.

Adolescents are known for their extreme ideals and emotions. I was no exception. But the unique perspectives and insights I gained through my experience during those years are still important to me today. The effects of the trauma I experienced have been resolved, but I am grateful that the positive lessons behind them have remained.

Whether your children are on the brink of adolescence with fluctuating moods, ideals, and emotions, or getting ready for the first grade, honor their experiences and take them seriously. The changes trauma brings into a young life can be transformative. You will be a tremendous help to your children when you listen to and acknowledge their transformation.

When traumatized children or their families tell me they believe their life has been ruined forever by what has happened to them, I say one thing: Life is more than the event. It's a part of it, but not all of it. As tragic and sad as a situation may be, it's not all of what life is.

To illustrate this idea, I ask children to imagine holding a book with their whole life written on the pages inside of it. Starting from the very beginning right up to today, I ask them to imagine the pages filled with every experience they've ever had. I instruct them to find where in their book they would find the frightening experience they've witnessed, heard about, or been through. I explain that this experience will be added to the many pages of memories they've had throughout their life. I invite them to turn to the pages where the frightening experience is written, and I help them learn how to skip to a happier section of their book when it feels too hard for them to face the trauma. I also give them the choice to close their book and put it away if they want to.

Traumatic experiences may take up a few lines in someone's life story, a few pages, or perhaps a whole chapter in the book. For others tragedy may be a central theme throughout their book, woven in and out of their young lives. Regardless of how many pages trauma fills, remind your children that it's not all of the book. It is a portion of it and no more.

Today I am privileged to be working with staff and students in Springfield, Oregon. I am honored to be among students and adults who know there is more to their school than the shooting that happened there. They realize Thurston High is much more than the trauma it has become famously associated with. One year after the shooting, wounds to the heart, mind, body, and soul were still mending and the pain continues to come in spasms for most, but like other schools victimized by gunfire, Thurston has their own life book filled with generations of memories, awards, and honors. The shooting will certainly take its place among the pages, permanently remembering the precious, innocent lives that were lost and all those who suffered injuries. But it will never be written over the past, and it need not detract from the future.

I am working with a team of caring adults from all walks of life who are committed to responding to the ongoing needs of area schools, staff, families, and all those in the community affected by the tragic shooting in Springfield. We are school staff, administrators, teachers, mental health professionals, grief counselors, law enforcers, media, legal advocates, court representatives, parents, clergy, and members of various community agencies, committed to working together to ensure ongoing support and healing through the days ahead.

As I sat in the first planning meeting with this committee, I was struck by the opportunity it presented us with. A chance to be an example to our kids. We recognize the work ahead cannot be done individually and must be done in relation to each other. We are committed to working as a team rather than independently or in competition with one another, not only because it is the right thing to do, but because it is also another opportunity for kids to see us model something very powerful. We are at another juncture where we can help kids regain trust in the world and show them the compassion that lives inherently in the people around them. We have the opportunity to show our children how caring people have chosen to come together in order to be of service to them. We can offer a view of the world that demonstrates kindness and compassion and renew their belief that good is stronger than evil.

The core issues that lie at the base of the wounded child's soul include the absence of hope and meaning in life. It's up to grown-ups to take action to help restore hope and meaning whenever and wherever possible. When this happens, children are given the welcome proof and understanding that once again more good can be seen than bad, more positive behaviors are evident than negative.

Adults have the sometimes daunting task of helping children through things they aren't sure how to get through themselves. As one group facilitator told school staff, who took extraordinary actions to save children's lives, "Thank you for being the grown-ups. Thank you for loving kids."

Hope must be continually renewed and experienced. It starts with us. Adults must step up to the plate in a variety of different ways and do what needs to be done with compassion and care. In the process, we are teaching the next generation how to do the same.

Children will continue to face the perils of living and we will continue to help them live through it. I am certain there will never be a shortage of caring adults, as long as there are adults who do their part now when life calls upon them to respond. And when they do, they are teaching children how to grow into adults who will know how to respond to their children and to the generations of children to come.

You can help your children write the next chapter of their lives with renewed hope and meaning. There's no better motivation than love.

References and

Resources

Allen, N. H. 1980. *Homicide: Perspectives on Prevention.* New York: Human Sciences Press.

Axline, V. M. 1969. *Play Therapy.* New York: Ballantine Books.

Bank, S. P., and M. D. Kahn. 1982. *The Sibling Bond.* New York: Basic Books.

Bowlby, J. 1985. *Attachment and Loss, Vol. III: Loss: Sadness and Depression..* NY: Basic Books.

———. 1980. *Attachment and Loss, Vol. II: Separation: Anxiety, and Anger Loss,* NY: Basic Books.

Davis, M., E. R. Eshelman, and M. McKay. 1995. *The Relaxation & Stress Reduction Workbook, Fourth Edition.* Oakland, Calif.: New Harbinger Publications.

Figley, C. R. 1985. *Trauma and Its Wake: The Study and Treatment of Post-Traumatic Stress Disorder.* New York: Brunner/Mazel.

———. 1986. *Trauma and Its Wake, Vol. II: Traumatic Stress Theory, Research, and Intervention.* New York: Brunner/Mazel.

———. 1988. Post-Traumatic Family Therapy. In *Post-Traumatic Therapy,* edited by F. Ochberg. New York: Brunner/Mazel.

———. 1989. *Helping Traumatized Families.* San Francisco: Jossey-Bass.

Figley, C. R. (editor). 1995. *Compassion Fatigue: Secondary Traumatic-stress Disorder from Treating the Traumatized.* New York: W.W. Norton.

Frankl, V. E., 1963. *Man's Search for Meaning: An Introduction to Logotherapy.* New York: Beacon Press.

Garbarino, J., E. Guttman, and J. W. Seeley. 1986. *The Psychologically Battered Child.* San Francisco: Jossey-Bass.

Garbarino, J. 1999. *Lost Boys: Why Our Sons Turn Violent and How We Can Save Them.* New York: The Free Press.

———. 1995. *Raising Children in a Socially Toxic Environment.* San Francisco: Jossey-Bass.

Gardner, G. E. 1971. Aggression and Violence: The Enemies of Precision Learning in Children. *American Journal of Psychiatry* 128(4): 445–450.

Herman, J. L. 1992. *Trauma and Recovery: The Aftermath of Violence from Domestic Abuse to Political Terror.* New York: Basic Books.

Jaffe, P., S. Wilson, and D. E. Wolfe. 1986. Promoting Changes in Attitudes and Understanding of Conflict Resolution Among Child Witnesses of Family Violence. *Canadian Journal of Behavioral Science* 18:356–366.

Janoff-Bulman, R. 1992. *Shattered Assumptions: Toward a New Psychology of Trauma.* New York: Free Press.

Jewett, C. L. 1982. *Helping Children Cope with Separation and Loss.* Harvard, Mass.: Harvard Common Press.

Krupnick, J. L. 1984. Bereavement During Childhood and Adolescence. In *Bereavement: Reactions, Consequences, and Care,* edited by M. Osterweis, F. Solomon, and M. Green. Washington, D.C.: National Academy Press.

Krupnick, J. L., and M. J. Horowitz. 1980. Victims of Violence: Psychological Responses, Treatment Implications. *Evaluation and Change* Special Issue: 42–46.

Lewis, K. G. 1988a. Symptoms as Sibling Messages. In *Siblings in Therapy: Life Span and Clinical Issues,* edited by M.D. Kahn and K.G. Lewis. New York: W.W. Norton.

———. 1988b. Young Siblings in Brief Therapy. In *Siblings in Therapy: Life Span and Clinical Issues,* edited by M. D. Kahn and K. G. Lewis. New York: W.W. Norton.

Lord, J. H. 1990. *No Time for Goodbyes: Coping with Sorrow, Anger, and Injustice after a Tragic Death.* Ventura, Calif.: Pathfinder Publishing.

Matsakis, A. 1992. *I Can't Get Over It: A Handbook for Trauma Survivors.* Oakland, Calif.: New Harbinger Publications.

Miller, A. 1981. *The Drama of the Gifted Child: The Search for the True Self.* New York: Basic Books.

———. 1983. *For Your Own Good: Hidden Cruelty in Child-Rearing and the Roots of Violence.* New York: Farrar, Straus, & Giroux.

———. 1986. *Thou Shalt Not Be Aware: Society's Betrayal of the Child.* New York: Meridian.

Mitchell, J. T. 1983. When Disaster Strikes: The Critical Incident Stress Debriefing Process. *Journal of Emergency Medical Services* 8(1):36–39.

Oaklander, V. 1988. *Windows to Our Children.* Highland, N.Y.: The Center for Gestalt Development.

Pynoos, R. S., and S. Eth. 1984. The Child as Witness to Homicide. *Journal of Social Issues* 40(2):87–108.

Pynoos, R. S., and S. Eth. 1985a. Children Traumatized by Witnessing Acts of Personal Violence: Homicide, Rape, or Suicide Behavior. In *Post-Traumatic Stress Disorder in Children,* edited by S. Eth and R. S. Pynoos. Washington, D.C: American Psychiatric Association.

———. 1985b. Developmental Perspective on Psychic Trauma in Childhood. In *Trauma and Its Wake: The Study and Treatment of Post-Traumatic Stress Disorder,* edited by C. R. Figley. New York: Brunner/Mazel.

———. 1985c. Interaction of Trauma and Grief in Childhood. In *Post-Traumatic Stress Disorder in Children,* edited by S. Eth and R. S. Pynoos. Washington, D.C.: American Psychiatric Association.

Staudacher, C. 1987. *Beyond Grief: A Guide for Recovering from the Death of a Loved One.* Oakland, Calif.: New Harbinger Publications.

Tedeschi, R. G., and L. G. Calhoun. 1995. *Trauma and Transformation: Growth in the Aftermath of Suffering.* Thousand Oaks, Calif.: Sage.

Terr, L. C. 1981a. "Forbidden Games": Post-Traumatic Child's Play. *Journal of the Amercian Academy of Child Psychiatry* 20:741–760.

———. 1981b. Psychic Trauma in Children: Observations following the Chowchilla School Bus Kidnapping. *American Journal of Psychiatry* 138(1):14–19.

———. 1989. Treating Psychic Trauma in Children: A Preliminary Discussion. *Journal of Traumatic Stress* 2(1):3–20.

———. 1990. *Too Scared to Cry: Psychic Trauma in Childhood.* New York: Harper & Row.

Van der Kolk, B. A., A. C. McFarlane, and L. Weisaeth (editors). 1996. *Traumatic Stress: The Effects of Overwhelming Experience on Mind, Body, and Society.* New York: Guilford Press.

Weaver, A. J., L. T. Flannelly, K. J. Flannelly, H. G. Koenig, and D. B. Larson. 1998. An Analysis of Research on Religious and Spiritual Variables in Three Major Mental Health Nursing Journals, 1991–1995. *Issues in Mental Health Nursing,* 19(3):263–276.

Wolfe, D. A., P. Jaffe, S. K. Wilson, and L. Zak. 1985. Children of Battered Women: The Relation of Child Behavior to Family Violence and Maternal Stress. *Journal of Consulting and Clinical Psychology* 53:657–665.

Wolfe, D. A., L. Zak, S. Wilson, and P. Jaffe. 1986. Child Witnesses to Violence Between Parents: Critical Issues in Behavioral and Social Adjustment. *Journal of Abnormal Child Psychology* 14:95–104.

Young, M. A. 1998. *Responding to Communities in Crisis: The Training Manual of the Crisis Response Team.* Washington, D.C: NOVA; and Dubuque, Iowa: Kendall/Hunt Publishing Co.

Helplines

1-800-CHILDREN
Confidential information and assistance for anyone concerned for children at risk for abuse. After hours, you may contact your local Department for Services to Children and Families, Department of Family Services, or State/local child abuse hotline.

The National Domestic Violence Hotline 1-800-799-7233 (twenty-four-hours a day); TDD: 1-800-787-3224.
Confidential information and assistance.

National Resource Center on Domestic Violence 1-800-537-2238;
TTY 1-800-553-2508; fax: 717-545-9456
Comprehensive information and resources.

Professional Organizations

Association of Traumatic Stress Specialists (ATSS)
7338 Broad River Road
Irmo, SC 29063
803-781-0017; fax: 803-781-3899; email: tidwel@netside.com
http://www.ATSS-HQ.com
ATSS is an international, nonprofit membership organization founded in 1989 to provide certification and professional educa-

tion to those actively involved in trauma response, treatment, management, and crisis organization. The association maintains an international list of skilled crisis responders, trainees, and therapists.

International Society for Traumatic Stress Studies
60 Revere Drive, Suite 500
Northbrook, IL 60062
847-480-9028
This is a organization for professionals from multiple disciplines interested in sharing advances in trauma research, theory, treatment strategies, and public policy. The organization has developed a resource pamphlet that can be sent out on request. Journal of Traumatic Stress is published for this organization four times a year by Plenum Press, 233 Spring Street, New York, NY 10013.

International Critical Incident Stress Foundation (ICISF, Inc.)
(a nonprofit foundation)
10176 Baltimore National Pike Unit 201
Ellicott City, MD 21042
410-750-9600; fax 410-750-9601

National Organization for Victim Assistance (NOVA)
717 D Street, N.W.
Washington, DC 20004
202-393-NOVA
Founded in 1975, NOVA is a private, nonprofit, umbrella organization working on behalf of victims of crime and other crises. The National Crisis Response Team (CRT) is part of NOVA's Division of Victim Services.
For more information: 202-232-6682
For victim assistance: 800-879-6682

MADD (Mothers Against Drunk Driving)
669 Airport Freeway, Suite 310
Hurst, TX 76053
Victim Line 1-800-Get-MADD

Audio Tapes

Davis, M., E. R. Eshelman, and M. McKay. 1987. *Progressive Relaxation and Breathing*. Oakland, Calif.: New Harbinger Publications.

Fanning, P. 1992. *Stress Reduction*. Oakland, Calif.: New Harbinger Publications.

Tools for Professionals

Coloring books for ages 4-10: Creative healing books for treating posttraumatic stress in children. Themes include: direct victimization, witness to violence, family violence, separation anxiety, and repressed memories. (To order call toll free 1-800-99- YOUTH.)

Alexander, D. W. 1991. *Something Bad Happened Series: Something Bad Happened; It Happened To Me; All My Feelings; I Can't Remember; Don't Go; The World I See.* Plainview, N.Y.: The Bureau for At-Risk Youth.

Journal-style stories for ages eleven to seventeen: Creative healing books for treating posttraumatic stress in adolescents. Themes include direct victimization, witness to violence, family violence, depression and suicidal thinking, identification of feelings, and survivors of homicide. (To order call toll free 1-800-99-YOUTH.)

Alexander, D. W. 1992. *Way I Feel Series: The Way I Feel; All My Dreams; It's My Life; It Happened in Autumn; When I Remember; In This House Called Home.* Plainview, N.Y.: The Bureau for At-Risk Youth.

Lagoro, J. 1993. *Life Cycle: Classroom Activities for Helping Children Live with Daily Change and Loss.* Tucson, Ariz.: Zephyr Press.

Pitcher, G. D., and S. Poland. 1992. *Crisis Intervention in the Schools.* New York: Guilford Press.

Books for Children

Beaudry, J., and L. Ketchum. 1987. *Carla Goes to Court.* New York: Human Sciences Press. (Grades K–6.)

Dutro, J. 1991. *Night Light: A Story for Children Afraid of the Dark.* New York: Magination Press. (Preschool–Grade 4.)

Galvin, M. 1988. *Ignatius Finds Help: A Story about Psychotherapy for Children.* New York: Magination Press. (Preschool–Grade 6.)

Hill, S. 1985. *Go Away, Bad Dreams.* New York: Random House. (Preschool–Grade 3.)

Mayer, M. 1968. *There's a Nightmare in My Closet.* New York: Dial Press. (Preschool–Grade 2.)

Moser, A. 1991. *Don't Feed the Monster on Tuesday: The Children's Self-Esteem Book.* Kansas City, Mo.: Landmark Editions. (Grades K–6.)

Palmer, P. 1995. *I Wish I Could Hold Your Hand: A Child's Guide to Grief and Loss.* San Luis Opispo, Calif.: Impact Publishers.

Sanders, C., and C. Turner. 1983. *Coping: A Guide to Stress Management.* Carthage, Ill.: Good Apple. (Grades 2–8).

Some Other New Harbinger Self-Help Titles

The Self-Esteem Companion, $10.95
The Gay and Lesbian Self-Esteem Book, $13.95
Making the Big Move, $13.95
How to Survive and Thrive in an Empty Nest, $13.95
Living Well with a Hidden Disability, $15.95
Overcoming Repetitive Motion Injuries the Rossiter Way, $15.95
What to Tell the Kids About Your Divorce, $13.95
The Divorce Book, Second Edition, $15.95
Claiming Your Creative Self: True Stories from the Everyday Lives of Women, $15.95
Six Keys to Creating the Life You Desire, $19.95
Taking Control of TMJ, $13.95
What You Need to Know About Alzheimer's, $15.95
Winning Against Relapse: A Workbook of Action Plans for Recurring Health and Emotional Problems, $14.95
Facing 30: Women Talk About Constructing a Real Life and Other Scary Rites of Passage, $12.95
The Worry Control Workbook, $15.95
Wanting What You Have: A Self-Discovery Workbook, $18.95
When Perfect Isn't Good Enough: Strategies for Coping with Perfectionism, $13.95
Earning Your Own Respect: A Handbook of Personal Responsibility, $12.95
High on Stress: A Woman's Guide to Optimizing the Stress in Her Life, $13.95
Infidelity: A Survival Guide, $13.95
Stop Walking on Eggshells, $14.95
Consumer's Guide to Psychiatric Drugs, $16.95
The Fibromyalgia Advocate: Getting the Support You Need to Cope with Fibromyalgia and Myofascial Pain, $18.95
Healing Fear: New Approaches to Overcoming Anxiety, $16.95
Working Anger: Preventing and Resolving Conflict on the Job, $12.95
Sex Smart: How Your Childhood Shaped Your Sexual Life and What to Do About It, $14.95
You Can Free Yourself From Alcohol & Drugs, $13.95
Amongst Ourselves: A Self-Help Guide to Living with Dissociative Identity Disorder, $14.95
Healthy Living with Diabetes, $13.95
Dr. Carl Robinson's Basic Baby Care, $10.95
Better Boundries: Owning and Treasuring Your Life, $13.95
Goodbye Good Girl, $12.95
Fibromyalgia & Chronic Myofascial Pain Syndrome, $19.95
The Depression Workbook: Living With Depression and Manic Depression, $17.95
Self-Esteem, Second Edition, $13.95
Angry All the Time: An Emergency Guide to Anger Control, $12.95
When Anger Hurts, $13.95
Perimenopause, $16.95
The Relaxation & Stress Reduction Workbook, Fourth Edition, $17.95
The Anxiety & Phobia Workbook, Second Edition, $18.95
I Can't Get Over It, A Handbook for Trauma Survivors, Second Edition, $16.95
Messages: The Communication Skills Workbook, Second Edition, $15.95
Thoughts & Feelings, Second Edition, $18.95
Depression: How It Happens, How It's Healed, $14.95
The Deadly Diet, Second Edition, $14.95
The Power of Two, $15.95
Living Without Depression & Manic Depression: A Workbook for Maintaining Mood Stability, $18.95
Couple Skills: Making Your Relationship Work, $14.95
Hypnosis for Change: A Manual of Proven Techniques, Third Edition, $15.95
Letting Go of Anger: The 10 Most Common Anger Styles and What to Do About Them, $12.95
Infidelity: A Survival Guide, $13.95
When Anger Hurts Your Kids, $12.95
Don't Take It Personally, $12.95
The Addiction Workbook, $17.95
It's Not OK Anymore, $13.95
Beyond Grief: A Guide for Recovering from the Death of a Loved One, $14.95
The Chemotherapy & Radiation Survival Guide, Second Edition, $14.95
An End to Panic: Breakthrough Techniques for Overcoming Panic Disorder, Second Edition, $18.95
Dying of Embarrassment: Help for Social Anxiety and Social Phobia, $13.95
The Endometriosis Survival Guide, $13.95
Grief's Courageous Journey, $12.95
Flying Without Fear, $13.95
Stepfamily Realities, $14.95
Coping With Schizophrenia: A Guide For Families, $15.95
Conquering Carpal Tunnel Syndrome and Other Repetitive Strain Injuries, $17.95
The Three Minute Meditator, Third Edition, $13.95
The Chronic Pain Control Workbook, Second Edition, $17.95
The Power of Focusing, $12.95
Living Without Procrastination, $12.95
Kid Cooperation: How to Stop Yelling, Nagging & Pleading and Get Kids to Cooperate, $13.95

Call **toll free, 1-800-748-6273**, or log on to our online bookstore at **www.newharbinger.com** to order. Have your Visa or Mastercard number ready. Or send a check for the titles you want to New Harbinger Publications, Inc., 5674 Shattuck Ave., Oakland, CA 94609. Include $3.80 for the first book and 75¢ for each additional book, to cover shipping and handling. (California residents please include appropriate sales tax.) Allow two to five weeks for delivery.

Prices subject to change without notice.

More New Harbinger Titles

SURVIVOR GUILT

A Self-Help Guide
Helps survivors make a realistic assessment of their role in a traumatic event and cope with how their feelings affect personal functioning ar'

TR

A G   **> Love Them**
Step   handle unre-
solv   hdrawal and
isola

I C

A H
The   iides readers
throu   one step at a
time.

WF

A H   **ildren**
Prov: l abuse, deal
with   d heal.
Item

Call   Mastercard
num   New Har-
bing   CA 94609.
Inclu   nal book to
cove   ise include
appr   ery.

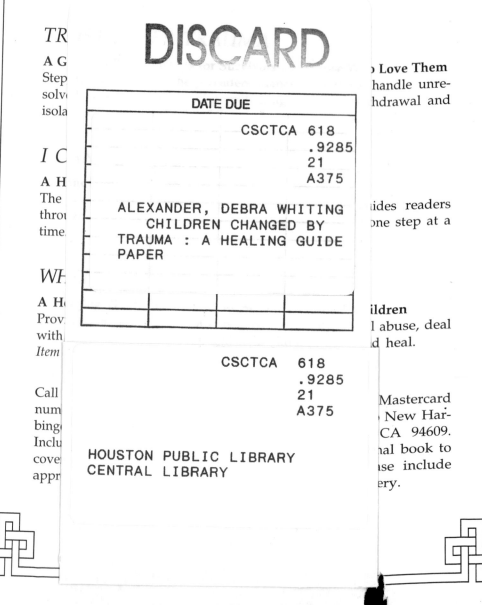